Heart
of
Persistence

Anastazia Ming

Contents

Acknowledgment

"I have to start by thanking my awesome husband, Steve. From the time this whole journey really came into play, you have been there. Whether it was to cheer me up, hear me cry, or just to be there. Thank you for being my special person."

"Without my parents, Tommy and Barbara, I never would have come this far.
They were my voice when I had none and fought for me through each battle like no other. I am forever grateful."

"They say a sister is your first friend and a second mother. I couldn't agree more. My sister Tammy, is truly one in a million. She has been there for me since the beginning and continues to be. I am blessed to have the sister that I do."

"Not too many people are as close to their nieces

as I am to mine. They have seen me at my worst but handled each situation with grace and attentiveness to my needs. To Raeann and Arianna, I say Thank you."

"To my children, Gianna, Frankie and Mia. What can I say, you have seen it all and lived through it with me. Sometimes, having to take a backseat for your own needs. Thank you for your patience while I wrote this book and for allowing me to be your Mama."

"To everyone else in my world, while you may not have weathered the battles with me, thank you for your kind words, and generosity throughout this journey. Your support is invaluable."

"Laughter is like a windshield wiper. It doesn't stop the rain, but allows us to keep going"

~anonymous~

Preface

Since the day I was born, I started fighting. Fighting to be healthy and live life normally that is. It wasn't until I was about eleven years old, I began to realize my fight. As you will see in this book, I encountered many, many concerning medical affairs of my heart. Not all of them were bad, but some put my life in jeopardy.

For forty-seven years, my life has been a roller coaster filled with ups and downs, twists and turns. It has even been upside down at times, involving myself and anyone that has been close to my heart. Through the years, science has come a long way. I am grateful for that. Who knows where I'd be if we still were operating the way we did back in 1974. It has always been my dream to live my life like a normal person. By normal I mean, walking a few blocks without getting winded or having the ability to run somewhere if I wanted to. The average person can do those things. I cannot. Tattoos, piercings and other works of art to the human body are a struggle for me to achieve. There is always a risk for me with infection. I can't even have routine dental work without being premedicated, or anything else done to my body for that matter.

The struggles of my life probably would have been much harder if there weren't laughs along the way. I truly believe laughter is what got me through my darkest times and hardest moments. As you will see from reading this book, I found humor in every situation or at least tried to. As I was writing this book, I rehashed all my memories. as I did a few times over the course of time. There were moments where I wasn't laughing at the time of the incident, but I did following it. In order to express my funny moments in this book to you as I see them, I put the word, (laughing) in parentheses.

The purpose of this book is to convey to the reader that life happens regardless. People will be people. There will be the great ones and there will be the not so great ones. Appreciate those that are in your corner and forget the ones that aren't. You can either grab your life by the balls and take control or you can bow down and let all your ailments bring you down. Each day brings new hope, purpose and meaning to life. I intend on fighting to the end and ensuring that no matter what or who is thrown my way, I handle it. This is my story.

Chapter one

Conditions of the Heart (1974-1999)

I believe every woman has a certain lifestyle they wish to live. Some are born to be mothers and by the time they are in their thirties, they have the whole soccer mom lifestyle. They drive a minivan, carpool with other moms, and get together during the day and the week for coffee. They do not care so much about their appearance, buying what is comfortable and what is on sale. Leggings and flat shoes are the most common. I want that lifestyle too, but not just only that lifestyle.

Tetralogy of Fallot: a rare condition caused by a combination of four heart defects that are present at birth. It was so long ago that I learned this term and had no clue what it meant, how I got it, or more importantly, how I could get rid of it. I think I was about eleven years old when I realized I was not like your average kid. Why did I turn blue when I stayed in a swimming pool too long or stayed outside in the cold for too long? Why couldn't I run down the block and not get out of breath like all the other neighborhood kids? I can remember having to hold my sister's hand when crossing the street, not because I did not know enough to stay away from a moving vehicle, but because I had to keep up with the pace at which she was walking! I would soon become familiar with what I grew up knowing as "my heart condition."

1987 would become the year this whole "heart condition" thing would become reality. Before this, I had all the symptoms above but never paid much attention. I would go for routine echocardiograms and just thought it was cool to be able to see what my heart looked like. I knew I had to see a special person called a cardiologist. You try saying that as a little kid! Little did I know at the time, that this would become a regular word in my vocabulary whenever I mentioned anything about my body. All I knew about this cardiologist was that she was a "special" doctor and liked to put these funny bulbs with wires all around my body (EKGS back in the 80s). For some reason, I liked smelling the alcohol preps that were used with the bulbs. This doctor would be my cardiologist until I was kicked out of the pediatric practice at age 21.

There was one visit, however, that was not so much fun. It was my yearly routine visit. I was twelve years old. I had an EKG first, followed by an echo. The doctor told my parents that they had to come to her office after my exam. I got dressed, and down the hallway, we went. My cardiologist as well as my parents looked very serious. There was not much smiling going on at that moment. The doctor explained to my parents that my latest echo now revealed some abnormalities and I had to undergo further testing for a more in-depth look at my heart. The next thing I knew, I had an appointment set up for a catheterization. Yet another word that I could not understand or pronounce!

It has been over 36 years since I had that test, so my memory is somewhat shaky. I do remember my cardiologist telling me there would be times it would feel like razors cutting me for a second. "Who tells a kid that???" I liked my cardiologist but – sheesh! I was so scared at that point. The hour-long test, or should I say what felt like ten hours, was brutal. Every minute I was asking my doctor if she was done. Even though my doctor was showing me how they can look at my heart, I was not impressed by seeing a long wire (catheter) being inserted into my groin and working its way up to my heart. I thought it was gross and wanted the whole experience to be over. The tiny inch scar left from that day would be the first of several scars to remind me of how just brave I can be.

The relief I would feel from knowing that the ordeal was over, would be short-lived. The test results came a few days later. The doctor called my parents. The findings of that test revealed that "it was time." "Time for what?" I asked. It was time to have my pulmonic valve replaced, as it had been deteriorating all this time. As I got older, I would often ask myself why the doctors did not choose to correct this valve at birth. I have been fortunate enough to meet a few people who were born with the Tetralogy of Fallot; all of whom had it corrected when they were infants. I must have asked at some point because I remember being told that the doctors wanted to wait until I was as old and as strong as possible before putting me through surgery. But still, why was I different from all the others? Was my condition more serious at birth than my peers?

As I write this, I can honestly say I don't remember the day of the surgery. I remember bits and pieces of the hospital stay after, however. It was the first time I had ever been away from my parents for so long. I was at the age when most kids start having sleepovers, but this is not what I had in mind. I was going to be sharing a room with a stranger, even though it would be another kid. The only one I have ever heard a cough, snore or ever fart while sharing a room to sleep with was my sister! (laughing)

I woke up the day after surgery in the Intensive Care Unit at a prestigious hospital in the city. My mother and father were there, smiling at me. My mother was patting my head and my father was patting my hand. I smiled back and tried to move. Well, a pain that I had never felt before shot through my arm like a knife! I did not know what was causing the pain, but it felt like my arm would fall off. I was told that my arm was probably sore from being in one position during the entirety of the 6-hour surgery. This pain would last for about two days and be worse than the pain I felt in my chest!

My grandmother came to visit me, afraid to sit on my bed. She thought she would hurt me. God rest her soul – I miss her. Anyway, ICU was great, however, the nurses came around constantly, asking me if I was ok and if I wanted anything. I had one nurse named Holly. If I could ever find her one day, I would thank her for taking such good care of me at night when my parents had to leave and go home.

During my hospital stay, I fell in love with the Tracey Ullman Show. I never cared for the show before, but it became my best friend during those first few days in ICU. It was all I had to amuse myself with when my parents were not around. As I said, laughter means so much. The one downside I did have – and again, I was twelve years old – was that my bed faced another bed directly across mine. The occupant of this bed was a boy who had to be a year or two older than me. Well, all he did was moan! I mean seriously, how could he have been in any more pain than me? To make it worse, he wore a hospital gown as well and I guess he did not like the blankets or sheets because they were rarely covering him. If you are familiar with Intensive Care, you know that you do not get out of bed for anything, including the bathroom! Therefore, you have a catheter inserted at all times throughout recovery No underpants are required! This encounter would be the first time my twelve-year-old self would see what male genitalia looks like. Luckily, my nurse realized it

14

too and closed his curtain. To this day, those images in my mind still haunt me, although maturation has slightly altered the memory to a more humorous one.

Once I survived ICU, I was moved to another unit. The only memories I have are of volunteers coming to take me to potholder-making class or ceramic tile ashtray class. I came home with a few handmade gifts for my parents. My parents did buy me a doll that I remember too. I remember because she talked. She would become my best friend for the week – her name was Pamela. No, I did not choose that name. That was the name the manufacturers gave to her.

Years later, I ended up Googling the doll because I was so curious. It turns out that this doll was manufactured during the eighties. I can purchase her on eBay if I like. As I type this, my older great-niece is two years old. I think I will buy it for her because I liked the doll so much and it gave me comfort when I needed it the most.

After eight days, I was discharged from

NYU. The ride home on the FDR hurt like hell. I felt every bump and turn my father made. There is one memory from that day that sticks in my mind. I lived on a street in the Bronx that held four apartment buildings. My father pulled up in front of the stoop to our apartment building and my parents helped me get out of the car. I started hearing clapping and cheering. When I looked up, I saw so many people with their heads out of their windows, chanting my name and clapping. The street was lined up with my neighbors standing on their stoops. Some even parked themselves in a lawn chair as if they were about to see a show! There was a huge white bed sheet hanging in front of my building that said "Welcome home." My mother's best friend had an apartment with three windows directly in the front of the building upon which the banner hung. Well, I felt like a celebrity! It was all about me at that point. I did not look like a celebrity, however. I was hunched over like an old lady, walking very slowly. The pain in my chest was so bad and I was so stiff that I could not stand up straight. I don't know how I ever made it up the steps of the stoop, but one thing was for sure... I was home.

The recovery from my first surgery was long and hard. I was about to turn 13 years old. Now being in my late forties, I can say that being thirteen is a hard time for a girl to go through. You're not considered a young child anymore, but yet not fully a teenager either. I now had a huge, ugly eight-inch scar in the middle of my chest that sat right in between what would shortly become fully developed breasts. I had no breasts then. Nothing on my body revealed me becoming a teenager. I was told that my heart condition had caused my body to not mature as quickly as it normally would have. Before the surgery, I weighed about sixty-five pounds. I think if anyone squeezed me hard enough, I would have snapped.

Everything would begin to change with me after the surgery, both physically and mentally.

Within three months, I had put on about

thirty pounds. My breasts started to develop. I remember my mother and her best friend being very excited about a gift I was about to receive from them – it was a bra. It looked more like a big bandage to me, and boy did it itch! I did not want these *boobs,* however, as you read on, you will see these boobs have their own story! I also got my period six months after that. Mentally, I changed too. I went to play with Pamela one night and became uninterested. I then pulled out my Barbie dolls, looked at them for a second, and put them away too. How could these toys that I once loved become so uninteresting to me, just like that? I suddenly started noticing boys and wanted to hang out with my older sister and her friends. She would often hang out in the local park or somewhere in the neighborhood, listening to music with her friends and doing things teenagers often do. I never cared about any of those things before the surgery. Forget about boys, I thought they were gross and disliked the way they acted and smelled. Now, I was intrigued by them.

As I stated earlier, becoming a teenager is hard. But you combine that with what I was going through – it just made it that much harder. Take going to school for instance. I was privileged to have a locker in junior high. No one else did in the seventh or eighth grades. But I did because I had two sets of textbooks each. One set to keep in school to transport to each class and another set I kept at home to do homework. The purpose of this was so that I would not have to carry around all that weight and put stress on my heart. My peers did not like that I was the only one with a locker and wanted to know what made me so special. Some even bullied me, taunting me about my heart condition and that I must be some sort of freak for having it. But I was special indeed. They were right about that. I tried my best to ignore the rude comments and poking fun. Another issue I had was gym class. We had uniforms for the gym. The t-shirt and shorts used to hang off of me. Now I had tiny bumps in the shirt and some butt cheeks in the shorts. I wasn't the only one that noticed. Before the surgery, I had nothing so I was often referred to as "Stacy no ass and Stacy no tits" by the male students in my school. Kids can be horrible! But after the surgery, my body started developing and the comments became less and less about having nothing and more like sexual harassment ones. Either way, I couldn't catch a break. I went to the neighborhood pool that following summer, and one girl came up to me because she noticed my scar and said, "Ewww, your chest looks gross!" Guess what happened next? I shoved her, straight into the ten-foot deep swimming pool, clothes and all. I am not going to lie – it felt good. It served her right for making fun of me. I didn't hurt her and I knew she could swim, so she got what she deserved. Sadly, it wouldn't be the last time my scar would make me get physical, but I will save that for another chapter.

It took me a while to be able to stand up straight after the surgery. Living in the Bronx, I would walk everywhere. But because I was slouched over, it was hard for me to get around. I went to one of my friend's birthday parties at her house soon after my operation even though I wasn't back on my feet fully at that point to physically go to a store and purchase a gift for her (online shopping did not exist back then). But still, I put ten dollars into a birthday card. When it came time to open the presents, she opened mine and announced to everyone, "ten dollars from Stacy, same thing as last year." I was so hurt and embarrassed, that I asked my friend's mother to use their phone. I called my father and begged him to come to pick me up. I only lived a few blocks away but could not walk back in my condition. My friend would later apologize after we got into an altercation in school and I expressed my feelings to her. It was the first time I would experience the truth that most people just don't care, and your problems are not theirs – no matter what your relationship is with them. Even the ones you wouldn't expect to react in a toxic way.

The following year, my family would move and I would start at a Catholic school for girls. Most of what I mentioned earlier would become painful memories of the past. No one knew me or my issues where I was going to be living, and no one that I went to school with previously would be in my new school. All these new girls knew was that I wore a scar with my uniform. But one thing remained the scar: I still had a heart condition. Having this disease, or whatever you want to call it, can impact a teenager's life both physically and emotionally. Every young lady wants to be beautiful and desirable to the opposite sex. At least I did.

Having a visible scar makes that difficult to accomplish. Turtle necks and crew neck shirts are not sexy looking to a teenage boy. But if I wore a low-cut v-neck shirt, guess what would also be revealed in addition to the little cleavage I had? I also had some scars right above my belly button. These were from tubes placed into my body during the surgery for fluid drainage. They looked like bullet holes and I took advantage of this by actually telling the people who asked about them that I got shot! Unfortunately, these scars did not accessorize well with a bikini. I would often feel so unattractive that I would cry. I could not wait for cold weather to come so that I could be all covered up. My body was still in the early stages of development; my teeth were crooked and I could not do anything about it because I still had so many baby teeth left due to the delay of my body maturing, adding yet one more insecurity to the list – I was a teenager with the body of a ten-year-old boy.

By the time I started dating boys, I had developed incredibly. There used to be a joke in my family about my breasts. It is said that Miracle-Gro was poured into my chest during surgery because I went from being flat to a C cup by the time I was 16, and then they did not stop growing! Although my boobs were there, I was still embarrassed to bear anything because of the scar. If a boy wanted to kiss me, I couldn't kiss back for more than a few seconds because I would be out of breath. Even though I had surgery to correct the valve, my body never seemed to fully function to its maximum capability. I still would get out of breath when running or being in cold air or kissing! Although it would appear that having a heart condition has nothing to do with having relations with the opposite sex, it did mentally and physically.

With every teenager comes the temptation to try new things. This could be sex, alcohol, drugs, etc. I was surrounded by friends that were all experimenting with pot and I was often called a "wuss" because I refused to share a joint with them. One, I found it gross that so many mouths could be on one joint (and Covid wasn't even a thing back then). But more importantly, my heart was weak, to begin with – what would happen to it if I started smoking pot? It was the same for smoking cigarettes. They cause damage to the normal person. So, imagine if I did those things? As for sex, that was something I experienced in my later teenage years. I already mentioned what kissing did to me, so you can guess how I would be during sex. Oxygen mask, please!!!! It's one thing to be out of breath after you're finished, but during? Not a turn-on (laughing).

Forget about all that. Just even doing something innocent was rough. I found it difficult to keep up with my friends with the dancing on the "Teen Nights" we used to attend. I would often have to sit down in the middle of the song because I was winded. Then there were fights. Never mind throwing punches around, I couldn't stand up long enough without losing my breath. Not that I was in the habit of fighting people, but I often had to defend myself from toxic individuals. I was scared to death of being punched in the chest and damaging my heart even more. Feeling this way made me a wuss, I guess, both appearance-wise and behaviorally. However, I did have someone in my corner: my sister – and for that, I am grateful that I have the sister that I do. She would often fight my battles for me and protected me like a mother bear would protect her cub. She even went after some girl who threatened me while being three months pregnant at the time with my niece. Tammy, my sister, is the reason I did not get my head beat in at times. I have witnessed from my teenage

25

daughter how cruel kids can be even when they pick on the average kid, and I am so glad that those days are over for me. Although, as you will read in future chapters, some people never mature and can continue to be cruel well into their adult life.

In 1996, I would have to go into the hospital again. Only this time, it was just for one night.

Since the age of 12, I have experienced swelling in my left foot that was more noticeable and uncomfortable in extreme temperatures. In hopes to address the cause, I went to see several vascular surgeons about this problem. One of them ordered an MRI. The MRI scan displayed that there was a vein and an artery in my groin crossing over one another, causing the swelling. It was mentioned that it may have been a result of the catheterization I had the year before. Regardless, sometimes the swelling became so bad, that I was unable to stand or walk – forget putting on a shoe.

One vascular surgeon I had consulted with

suggested putting in a stent to open up my blood flow because I was not receiving enough circulation. Here we go again with the razor cutting and having me stay awake for it! At least they did give me a sedative to relax me. I guess it did something because I don't remember the doctor talking to me afterward.

I was in the recovery room and my mother was apologizing to me. "For what" I had asked.

She replied by saying, "for putting you through all of this and not even having it work." I did not know what she was talking about so she explained. As it turns out, the stent procedure was not successful. The vascular surgeon felt the stent could have the potential to move and therefore could potentially result in a blood clot forming. I did not know whether to be more upset that the swelling would not be disappearing or that I had gone through that for nothing. The surgeon told my parents as well as me that the only other alternative was to make an incision alongside my abdomen and down my leg to have my vein removed from lying on top of my artery. It was major surgery. I said, "no way!" and my parents agreed. I was already scared enough. The foot swelling was a nuisance but not life-threatening. I could live with it even though it had its issues. To this day, my foot still swells, making it painful at times. I still struggle with finding comfortable shoes to wear; my foot does not look attractive being squashed and puffy in a sandal and it is so hard to wear any tight shoes. It's bad enough that I can't flaunt my chest in a sexy way but my foot too? I have already mentioned how girly I am, so you can imagine how frustrating this was for me since I love shoes. It does, however, help to make my kids feel guilty when I am at the sink for too long doing dishes and my foot starts to swell, inspiring them to *sometimes* offer to take over. I said sometimes, right?

Chapter 2

Gianna Marie (1999-2003)

So, by now, you have an understanding of what it was like for me growing up with the Tetralogy of Fallot. I was able to function daily with minimal complications, though I adapted and it progressed into more of a mental thing at this age than a physical one. Having my first child would be the first time since my surgery that my heart condition would interfere and complicate things once again.

When I was young, doctors told my parents that there would be several complications with my ability to become pregnant and carry one with my heart. I was already going to have a hard enough time carrying a pregnancy to term with the weight and stress on my body, let alone giving birth. In other words, there was a chance I would not be able to have children. But this was revealed in the early '80s. Much was still to be known. Fast forward to the late 90s, and even though I had a heart condition present, this assumption had vanished by the time I was twenty-four.

In the summer of 1998, I became pregnant with my daughter. I was twenty-three years old and unmarried. I remember the day I found out. I was petrified. I thought about everything the doctors had said about me being pregnant. I thought I was either going to die or my child would. I hid the pregnancy from my family for three months, telling only my boyfriend (who is now my husband!). I think back now and realize that this was stupid because I put myself and my unborn child at risk. Even though my body was handling it normally and with no complications, I did not know that – I lived in a constant state of worry. In the eighth week, I thought I had miscarried. I began having brown discharge, which to me meant I was bleeding, and this was not good at all. To make matters worse, I was away at a friend's house while this was happening. My friend had no more knowledge than I did. Blood on its own is a risk for me to begin with because I am at a higher risk than the average person for a bacterial infection. However, I do believe God works in mysterious ways because an obstetrician opened an office next door in the building where I worked. He was new to the area and was doing consults at no charge, so I went to see him. He told me my pregnancy was very much viable and what I was experiencing was the baby implanting itself in my wound to stay! That was the first time I got to see my baby's heartbeat. At that moment, I knew this pregnancy was a blessing and nothing meant more to me than having this baby. I knew I would have to eventually tell my family as I would be "showing" soon and wanted to have this baby. I had also been told by the doctors that if I was going to try to have children, I should have them at a young age. My heart would not be as strong the older I got. So, as I was in my twenties and was able to conceive, I was determined to see this through at all costs.

As it turns out, Tammy was the first one to find out. I attended a party she was throwing in her apartment for one of her friends. Noticing my adamancy to not consume alcohol, my sister questioned why I wasn't drinking and then proceeded to poke me in the stomach and tell me I was getting fat. (laughing). All of a sudden, she frowned. She did not have to say anything anymore. The look on her face told me she knew. All she kept saying was "Oh my God." She then cried to her friend out of fear for me and my health. She held it in for a week and then told me it was time to tell my parents. My sister was concerned about what this pregnancy would do to my heart.

I have stated earlier that Tammy has always been there for me – this time was no different. The day came to tell my parents about the pregnancy. We had planned to have dinner, with my sister, my parents, and me, and I had every intention of attending. However, due to an argument with my boyfriend over this and other issues, I never showed up because I was on the verge of breaking up with him. So, Tammy was left to be the bearer of the news. I am sure she would have liked to kill me at that moment. My family has a long history of having babies and getting married afterward – it is just how it goes. So, the way my sister tells me the story of what happened goes something like this:

She tells them I am pregnant. My mother gets upset and asks, "How could she?" My sister then says, "You did it, I did it and every other female in this family did it. Why should she be any different?" Then my mother says, "But she has a heart condition." And Tammy says, "Well, she is still human." My mother called my cellphone and just whispered "Come home." I thought about running away. Nevertheless, in all seriousness, there was a week of upset, anger, and disappointment. I got yelled at by both my mother and father at first, and then it turned into concern for me and my baby.

By the time everyone knew I was pregnant, I had already been done with the first trimester.

Now I was starting to show. I also started filling out all areas of my body. I found this to be funny because I was always so skinny. My breasts became triple D's which, as you know from previous chapters, had increased in size over time. My mother took me shopping for maternity clothes and we purchased maternity bras in size E. I never even knew that they went up that high! It was so hard to tell where my chest ended and where my belly started. I was just round and could not see my shoes. My boyfriend proposed to me during my third trimester also. It was a cold night in February when he did it. We were sitting outside in a park near his house, eating ice cream! I said yes, belly and all.

As for my heart... well like I said earlier, I was kicked out of the pediatric practice at age 21. I never retained a new cardiologist after that, thinking I was going to be fine after that surgery in 1987. Up until this point, I only had routine visits, EKGs, and echocardiograms, all of which would show the same thing: I was fine and there was no change. I knew being pregnant was different, however, and I had to find a new cardiologist. I did find one and on my first exam; he was so laid back about my condition and being pregnant that I got the impression there was nothing to worry about. Was everything I had been told a lie or just some misinformation because there was not enough research on women with the Tetralogy of Fallot and pregnancy? Or maybe science made huge strides in research and now you can just pop some sort of pill and be fine? Either way, I made sure I followed up with him during my pregnancy, ensuring that neither myself nor my baby was in any danger of complications as a result of my condition.

There was one visit in my third trimester where my cardiologist stated to me that he would like to perform a fetal echocardiogram on me to make sure my baby's heart was ok. I was alarmed by this and questioned him on it. To my knowledge, I had a heart condition, but it was just a fluke thing that happened at birth. It is not considered hereditary like breast cancer or something else of that nature. The doctor responded by telling me it isn't considered hereditary, but they take all precautions. So, I had this test and, although I already knew what to expect about echocardiograms, this one was a little different. Normally, the technician would move the probe around my chest cavity to get images of my heart. But in this case, the probe had to be placed below my breasts to get clear images of my baby's heart. This made for an extremely uncomfortable position for me. A piece of the table that I was lying on had to be removed for my stomach to fit. Then my breasts had to be lifted to get the probe to the baby's heart. I've already mentioned how endowed I had become. Each breast was so big that the technician had to place my breast on top of the probe to get to the area she needed to be near. She had to push, or should I say ram the probe, into my skin to try to get a clear image. Mammography is less painful! It wasn't a pleasant experience but in the end, it was all worth it! There was an advantage to all of this. Because the fetal echo is very much like a sonogram, I got pictures from it. So, it was like having another sonogram but with a chance to get more photos at a different angle. To my excitement, my daughter's heart was just fine! Watching her tiny heartbeat away in her little body was so amazing and beautiful, and I will never forget it – I was in awe.

Gianna Marie was born two weeks before her due date. I was spending the night at my boyfriend's house because I wasn't going to be able to see him for a few days. I was going to be leaving for Tammy's house. My sister lived closer to the hospital and we were taking all precautions. I needed to get to the hospital as quickly as possible when the time came in case of any issues. As it turns out, I never made it to her house. I woke up the next morning at my boyfriend's house and felt like I had peed a little bit in my underwear. It wasn't like a full pee that one would normally take, or enough to describe what I had heard about a pregnant woman's water breaking, but just enough to make me feel wet. This went on for another hour or two. I would feel a trickle then it would stop. I called the obstetrician and he told me it sounded like I was leaking amniotic fluid. He did not want to take any chances with me having a dry birth, so I was advised to go to the hospital the next morning to be induced. I was 2 weeks away from my due date, so this was reasonable. I called the entire family, "Get ready! We're having a baby!"

The next morning came and my family and I ran around like crazy! Everyone was so nervous; I had so many mixed emotions. I was excited that I was finally going to be a mother and have that baby that I was told I might never have. I was also frightened by what could happen to me as it was a risk. But no matter what, I was going to see this through.

I arrived at the hospital and was hooked up to every wire possible. There were so many people coming in and out of my room, asking me the same questions over and over. I was told that as the induced drug, Pitocin, started to work, I would start feeling some pain from the contractions at some point and that it would increase as time went on. The nurse asked me if I wanted an epidural when the time came. Absolutely! I was advised of the risks – blah blah blah. I started to feel some discomfort while the epidural was inserted, but once in place, it began to work. Truth be told, I didn't feel anything after that! There was even a mention of them decreasing the epidural effect because it was working so well that I wouldn't be able to push from not feeling anything. I told them, "Don't you worry! I will push!" The pushing lasted for about two hours. I had five people cheering me on: my boyfriend, my mother, my sister, the doctor, and a medical student named Suki – she was a very friendly Asian woman who kept cheering, "C'mon Stacy! I see a baby head!" (laughing)

Twelve hours after arriving at the hospital, my beautiful daughter, Gianna Marie, was born. She was the most beautiful baby I had ever seen. I say this not because she is mine, but some do come out looking all scrunched up and red. Not my Gianna though. She was beautiful, and to this day, she still is. I will never forget the first time she looked at me and we locked eyes. I knew we were bonded forever. I also felt like a hero. I had just accomplished what some doctors believed I would not be able to. The thought of that alone was enough to fill my weak heart with some strong happy emotions. I was able to conceive, go through labor and have a beautiful baby, all while having a heart condition. Maybe I could be like everyone else. Just gotta believe and fight. This would be the first hurdle of a few where I beat the odds.

Nevertheless, I am not gonna lie, the first few days at home with my new baby were stressful. I tried to breastfeed my daughter, but as big as my breasts had gotten, I could not. After two days of trying and being so engorged, I decided to stop. Gianna was crying because she was not receiving enough milk and I was running a fever from the engorgement. I felt like a failure at that point. All I ever wanted was to become a mom and do all of the things that I believed mommies did. I also had an episiotomy while giving birth – I was hurting. Because of this, I could not walk for a week, I had to crawl on the floor and pull myself up to the closest thing I could get to stand. Once I got over that hump, things began to fall into place and I had a routine; the rest became smooth sailing.

The next few years of my life would become quiet and just "normal." I stayed home with my daughter for a year, tending to her. I went back to work eventually and found a lovely woman to watch my daughter who, conveniently, only lived a block away from where my job was. My life had new meaning and purpose which is what I dreamed of having for so long. I loved it. I went to work, came home, and catered to my fiancé and my daughter. My job was short-lived, however. One morning, I wore a blazer with a tank top underneath it my – scar was showing since the cut of the top was a few inches above the cleavage point – and I was standing outside my boss's office waiting to ask her something. Another coworker, whom I wasn't a fan of due to her rude and ignorant behavior, was also standing there. She stared at me for a few seconds and then said, "Who cut you all up?" I felt my blood boil and my heart race. What adult is that rude and ignorant to ask that? I wanted to punch her. "What did you just say to me, you ignorant ass?" She clocked a fist, so I did too. Just then, my boss came rushing in between us. "You both are put on suspension for disorderly conduct and will be written up for this!" She barked. I barked right back. "Forget all that. Don't waste your time. I quit! Cuz if I don't, there will be another fight between me and her."

With that, I grabbed my stuff, walked out, picked up my daughter, and called Steve. I refused to deal with the cruelty of some humans. I was born fighting and always will as long as someone mistreats me. I found a new job a month later, but this time I was only working part-time. I just was missing one thing. Although we were engaged, the mention of marriage did not come up too often. I wanted to be married since we shared a daughter and I was in love. We were struggling to get ahead financially, however, but as long as we were all under one roof – happy and healthy, the marriage could wait.

We eventually ended up getting married, finally tying the knot three years after I was proposed to. I was starting to think about having another baby and wanted to not be unwed with two kids. One more child, however, would complete the puzzle, and I wanted to complete it. My first pregnancy had no complications heart-wise or with anything else, so why not? We had a beautiful wedding with about 200 of our closest family and friends. Gianna was even one of our flower girls. My life would remain unchanged except that I was a married woman now.

After a while, I realized that I was going to need a job with medical benefits. Having this heart problem meant frequent trips to the doctor's office as well as expensive testing. God forbid if I required another surgery. My part-time job offered no benefits and I could no longer afford to pay out of pocket for the individual plan I had purchased to cover me while I was pregnant.

I applied for a job with several companies but there was one in particular that I was interested in. It was for a cardiology group located near my mother-in-law's house and also near my daughter's babysitter's home. Not only would I be able to get Gianna to the babysitter, but it would give me a chance to learn everything there is to know about cardiology! It was a win-win situation!

I faxed over my resumé and a few days later I received a call from the manager of the cardiology group. She liked my resumé and was interested in setting up an interview with me. I met with her and explained all about my heart condition and my experience with it. I told her that I would be enthusiastic and proficient with my work because I had a passion for what this company provided to its patients and respect for its mission. I ended up getting the job and learned several things along the way. As part of my duties, I often had to pull patients' medical records to support medical necessities – not that I abused my position and read people's files, but sometimes I had to search in reports to find something that supported the diagnosis. After some time reading medical jargon, I began to learn a few things. I am proud to say that I stayed there for fifteen years, up until I became disabled. However, that's a story for another chapter!

Speaking of learning new things about cardiology, I learned much more than I ever knew from having a heart problem myself. For instance, there is a difference between having a heart defect versus having heart disease. I never knew that vascular problems were linked to cardiology, even though I saw that vascular surgeon when I was younger for the stent. Now that I was working with insurance companies, and submitting medical records, I would find myself reading the echocardiogram and nuclear reports. I tried to educate myself and, in some small way, tried to find a cure for my problem. Although I do know today that this is not possible, I still found it all intriguing and wanted to know more. As I write this today, I can confess I am still learning new things.

My life remained pretty quiet during this time and then in December 2003, I found out I was pregnant again. We hadn't been actively trying but weren't exactly preventing it either.

Finding out about this pregnancy made me overcome with joy! My first pregnancy was so unlike what the doctors had predicted. I was never on bed rest, I only gained 20lbs and, more importantly, there were no heart issues. This time I was in a better place mentally, emotionally, and financially. I was a married woman, we had a place of our own and I was still young. Plus, I already had medical benefits. Like all the doctors had told me, "have 'em' young." I also was going to be giving birth in the summer, unlike my daughter who was born in the winter. It would be a whole new experience that I was looking forward to. Christmas was around the corner and I managed to keep my pregnancy to myself, and my husband for three weeks. I was going to make my announcement at Christmas dinner. I purchased two ornaments, one for my mother's house and one for my mother-in-law's house. It was an ornament of a house with four windows, each had our names on it with the word "baby" and our last name displayed in the last window. This is how I was going to tell the family. Both announcements went fantastic! The grandmothers were overjoyed as were the other family members. There was not as much fear or concern this time since we had been through this previously and were successful. We could all relax a little.

Chapter 3

(2003-2006) Frankie Thomas

For my second pregnancy, I wanted to do things a little differently. There was so much concern and precautions with my first child that it was hard to enjoy. Now that I knew I was capable of carrying a pregnancy to term, I was gonna take it easy with the second.

I decided to look for a new obstetrician. My first one was awesome, but I did not want to have to travel to the city to give birth. I had heard so many stories of women not making it to the delivery room on time and giving birth in a cab or something like that. Besides, I lived close to Greenwich Hospital. It was the "elite" of hospitals. I was going to feel like I was in a hotel and I was excited. I chose an all-female obstetrics group. I had to meet with each one because they were always on call for one another and no one knew for sure who would be doing the delivery.

The one thing I did not want, however, was to have a midwife deliver my baby. Not that I feel midwives are not competent, I just thought that with my heart condition, I needed a medical doctor to oversee things. This group understood that and assured me I would have one of the MDs would deliver my baby when the time came.

Going through the summer months would be more difficult than I had anticipated. The hot weather made my feet swell so much that I could barely walk at times. My breasts increased in size and I just became round, waddling to wherever I had to go. Just like my first pregnancy, I could not wait to find out what I was having, and, unsurprisingly, I was overjoyed when I found out I was having a boy. We already had a little girl and now a boy would make my family complete. There hadn't been a boy born into our family in over twenty years, so I wanted to announce it specially. However, gender reveals were not a thing then, so I went with the first thing I thought of. I had the technician print me out a sonogram photo of just the baby's genitalia. She put the cursor on it for the pic. I showed the picture to my mother the next day. "Is that what I think it is?" I nodded. At some point in the pregnancy, I had the same fetal echocardiogram as I did with my first. Just like his older sister, the baby boy's heart looked great on the test!

In theme with his older sister, my son came 2 weeks before his due date, only this time there would be no inducing. I was at my parent's house. We had just gotten back from dinner and I was spending the night. Well, I would never get to sleep in my old bed because my water broke that night. I was sitting down on my parent's couch, watching TV with my father. I felt some wetness in my underwear, went to the bathroom, and noticed speckles of pink on my underwear. "It won't be long now!" I told my mother what just happened and then went back to the couch to watch tv with my father. As I sat down, I heard a "pop" and then water came rushing out of my shorts and down my legs. It was a mix of clear and pink. My father's first reaction was to jump up and shout, "Get off my couch!" The couch was only a couple of weeks old, you see, and it took about eight months to get to them as it traveled from Italy. My mother was running around like a lunatic, chanting, "Oh my God, oh my God!" (We had just gotten back from dinner and she may have had a few cocktails). She called my obstetrician and was talking to the doctor in such a panic that my doctor asked to put me on the phone. I explained what had happened and the doctor told me I was calmer than my mother! She gave me the option to wait until I started having contractions and when they were several minutes apart to leave for the hospital, or I could go to the hospital right away if I was uncomfortable with having a heart condition. I chose to go to the hospital at that time. My mother called my fiancé and he drove over to my mother's house to pick me up as well as my anxious mother. The contractions started coming while we were en route. It only took about twenty minutes to get to the hospital but the contractions were coming on strong. I yelled at my fiancé to drive faster. I did

51

not want to have this baby in the car on a highway, and I was also afraid of my heart not being monitored.

We arrived at the hospital and I was sent to labor and delivery right away. I was asked if I wanted an epidural, which I gladly told them to do. The next few hours would consist of pain and exhaustion. The epidural never completely took effect and I was hurting. I was also so tired as it was now the middle of the night. My fiancé fell asleep in a chair and my mother kept stroking my hair. We called the anesthesiologist several times. Once he did arrive, he told me I was at my maximum dosage for epidural and he could not administer any more to me. I told him I was in a lot of pain. Though he did not understand how that could be, he told me there was nothing else he could do. I respect doctors and all but when it comes to pain, I am an expert as well. I think he needed more medical training. To this day, I don't think I have met someone (and I have met many anesthesiologists in my lifetime) that was as rude and incompetent as he. But in the end, pain and all, I saw that labor to the end. I often cringe when I hear women say, "You want to know pain? Try having a baby." I say this to them: "No, you want to know REAL pain, have open-heart surgery. Giving birth can't even compare."

My Frankie was born at almost 3 a.m. I was exhausted. I had been pushing for about four hours. My eyes were bloodshot and I endured tearing when I was delivering him. I refused an episiotomy after my experience with Gianna, but he was worth it! At last, I had a son! My life felt complete. I had one girl and one boy. Again, something that my family nor the doctors thought could be possible. I beat the odds, not once but twice. I fell in love with my son from the very start.

Life with two kids, instead of just one, was a whole new world! I was used to napping when my daughter did or relaxing after she went to bed. Now it seemed like when one of them was content and could amuse themselves, the other one needed me, and then vice versa. God forbid they took a nap at the same time! It seemed like all I did was pump breast milk as well, even though I had to avoid alcohol. I could have relied on the "pump and dump" method, but I didn't want to take any chances. Plus, I was determined to breastfeed this time. My breasts were twice the size of my son's head, so how could milk not come out of them? I had to hold my breast up while he nursed or I might have suffocated him! I rented a breast pumping machine from the hospital. This thing was powerful! After I pumped each time, my nipples were about the same size as wire nuts! I pumped so others could feed him at times and give me a break. Also, I wasn't in the habit of whipping out a boob in public, and not getting paid for it? No thanks! Frankie was breastfed for three months, right up until I returned to work. For the first week or two, I had to wear those breast pad things in my bra because I would leak sometimes when my milk was drying up. A wet work shirt would be embarrassing!

My chest eventually decreased a little bit after my milk had dried up. However, my size remained a triple D! This was way too much breast for me to handle! I am only five feet and two inches tall and weigh about 120lbs (at the time, ahem). Each breast weighed so heavily on me that I experienced back, shoulder, and neck pain. I had to see a chiropractor to give me adjustments just so that I could function daily. I reached a point where I couldn't take it anymore. I was in so much pain, constantly having to lie down to give my neck and back some relief. Nothing looked cute on me because I had to purchase tops that were two sizes bigger to accommodate my chest. They just made me look bigger all around. And forget about wearing a bikini! My mother would laugh at me when I was at the beach or pool and say I looked like a stripper. My boobs are 100% real, but they were so big that they looked fake. Yes, it was time to do something about these bad boys! (laughing).

I began looking into breast reduction surgery. I had heard that some insurance companies will pay for the surgery itself. I also heard that it is much more painful than breast augmentation. Regardless, I wanted to have the surgery. But once again, my heart condition was an issue. I made an appointment to see my cardiologist and, to my surprise, he told me that I should be fine and experience no complications from having a breast reduction. I was overjoyed. I went to consult with a plastic surgeon that someone had recommended. She explained the whole process and told me there would be minimal scarring, but the surgery would leave some type of mark. For once, I did not care about the scar. I already had a huge one on my chest, so what difference did it make if I added two more small ones? I wanted to look good in both a tight top and a bikini top! I also needed to be able to stand up straight once again – be able to lift my kids, and not feel any pain. (laughing).

Dealing with the insurance company was a nightmare. At first, my request for coverage was denied. They considered it "cosmetic." And not "medically necessary." I asked the plastic surgeon's office what I could do about this. They replied by telling me I needed as much medical history and documentation as possible to support the pain I was feeling as a result of being well endowed. So, I requested all of my medical records from the chiropractor and sent them over to the insurance company. Yet I was denied again. This time it was a "lack of clinical documentation." My primary care physician recommended I see a neurologist. So I did. I was referred to a petite doctor with a very small chest. I mentioned the pain I had been feeling and all was fine. It was when I told her I was trying to have breast reduction surgery that the doctor's mood changed. She became somewhat agitated and told me that she was not going to see me for one or two visits and then write a letter of medical necessity for me if that is what I was here for. Basically, in not so many words, she was implying that I was using her. My first reaction was to get up and walk out. It shouldn't matter my reason for being there. Patients should be treated with respect and courtesy regardless of

57

what you may think I'm there for. A doctor should remain professional. However, I needed her documentation to support my necessity claim. So, I took a deep breath and told her my pain was real and the only solution was to have surgery, but if she wanted to try some methods, then I was all for it. Even though this lady was a doctor, no one knew my body better than I and I knew nothing was going to work. However, the more medical documentation where everything else failed, the better! The doctor's first method was to inject me with Cortisone shots to relieve the pain. Maybe her real reason for giving me a hard time was to get as many visits and therapies out of me as she could to milk my insurance company. But did I accuse her? No. She injected several shots into my back, each was excruciating. I was in tears by the time she was done, but I had to come back and see the doctor the following week for another treatment. I went back to her that following week and explained that we would no longer be doing the injections. While they took my pain away, I had soreness in my back for three days after being injected. I explained to the doctor that while this solved one problem, it created another. And what was I supposed to do? Keep getting injected for the rest of my life or until my breasts fall off? At least this time she agreed.

The doctor suggested trying something else: an ECG test. So, there I sat for forty minutes, getting poked in my wrist only to find out that I had carpal tunnel syndrome, which I already knew. The doctor finally advised setting me up for an MRI of my neck and back. Did it take several visits to order this? Now, again, who is using who? As I said, my insurance company was billed each time and she was getting paid. But they're not too bright themselves. All of these visits and tests probably amount to the same cost as breast reduction itself, give or take. They just created more paperwork for themselves. Nevertheless, this would be the smartest thing the doctor did in all the time I spent with her.

I returned to the doctor's office after having

the MRI. The doctor was retrieving the medical report of my MRI off of her fax as I walked in. She took one look at the report, her mouth dropped, and then she looked at me. Her exact words were, "Wow. You weren't kidding. You are in a lot of pain. You have five herniated discs between your neck and your back." I replied by saying, "I told you my pain was for real." The doctor smiled at me and told me that she would have her letter of medical necessity ready for me to pick up the next day along with all of her documentation. I was overjoyed. I was hoping this would finally be exactly what I needed to have the surgery because I had no other tricks up my sleeve.

Once I had the neurologist's letter of medical necessity, I wrote my letter to my insurance company, detailing all of the pain and struggles I had been going through as a result of my breast size. My letter was three pages worth. I told them how much stress it was causing on my heart weight-wise, among other things. A few weeks later, I received a letter from the insurance company, authorizing approval to pay for the surgery. I had succeeded, finally. My persistence paid off. I went back to see the plastic surgeon and made a date for the surgery.

In 2006, the day came for the surgery and I was excited. My husband, however, was sad. He cupped my breasts in his hands, "goodbye my friends." (Isn't that a typical man for ya!) (laughing). Most women get excited about breast implants, I was excited to be losing my breasts! I don't remember too much from that day. I know the room they had put me in looked more like a hotel than a hospital room, so that was nice. I woke up from the surgery and my chest was completely covered in bandages. So much so that I looked flat! I thought to myself, "Oh God! What have I done?" The surgeon explained they were wrapped very tightly to avoid bleeding. She later told me that she had taken three pounds of breast tissue out of my breasts. It did not sound like much, but when I stood up I felt the weight off my shoulders, literally.

The recovery was a little bit harder than I had

expected. It would take about two weeks before I could resume normal activities, such as lifting or driving. I could not take a shower because the water could not hit my chest directly. Now and then, a sharp pain would rip through my chest, making me jolt. There were times I wished I hadn't done this but my neck and back still felt better than they ever had.

On my first day back to work, I went without a bra. I could never have done that before the surgery. I always had to wear a heavy-duty underwire bra for support. I work with a bunch of women and all of them knew I was having the surgery. Most women don't like to reveal they have implants, but hey, I was proud to say I had to cut mine off because they were so big! The morning that I returned to work, all eyes were on me, my chest in particular. I was told I looked much thinner, more proportionate – things like that. I felt good.

The summertime was approaching and it was time to go bathing suit shopping. I couldn't wait! For the first time since I was a teenager, I was going to try on a bikini. I always had to wear one-piece bathing suits that were too big for every other area of my body other than my chest. I must have purchased about ten bathing suits that day, including a Louis Vuitton suit. I treated myself. I couldn't wait to flaunt it and my two new and improved puppies.

As you read on, you will see that I would come to regret having this surgery in some ways. I had complications because of it, but for now, I will continue with the next journey that came after this.

Chapter 4

These Things Just Happen (2006-2009)

My life for the next two years continued as normal as possible. My heart was stable and I had nice boobs. I was a wife and mother of two beautiful children. We were starting to think of purchasing a home as we had begun to outgrow our apartment. I loved where I lived but wanted a house with a backyard and stairs. The houses in our neighborhood were either too pricey or just not what we were looking for.

In August of 2006, I found out I was pregnant with our third child. Now we had to move! We could get by in the apartment with two children, but not with three! I wanted to find an area that we could afford while getting a decent size house and, most importantly, have Gianna attend a school that was comparable to the school district she was currently in. Frankie would eventually be going to school as well. We needed to look further up the line, however, for more affordable options. I would just have to sacrifice. I spent the next few weeks reading Pregnancy magazine and looking at real estate listings online. With my heart condition, the obstetrician felt it was a good idea to be evaluated by a perinatologist. Part of that evaluation included a transvaginal ultrasound. I went to the hospital at eight weeks to have this done. My father came with me for support and to drive me. The tech performing the test was a young lady in her twenties. She had me lie down and proceeded to begin the exam. As soon as she placed the probe inside of me, she withdrew it and said she was going to have the doctor come in to take a look. As soon as she said that, I knew something was wrong. It was only about a minute or two before the doctor came into the room, but it felt like an eternity. The doctor finally came in and performed her exam, all while I was craning my neck so hard to watch what was going on the screen. After a few minutes, the doctor withdrew the probe and told me she had some bad news. My baby, or fetus as the doctor had described, had stopped growing at seven weeks. That was just the week prior! She went on to explain that sometimes these things happen and they have no answers. I cried like a baby while getting dressed and walking out into the waiting room. My father saw the look on my face and knew I had lost the baby. He tried to console me, but I just didn't want to hear it. The doctor offered me two options: I could come back to the hospital in the next few days and have a D and C to clean out my uterus, or wait it out and let the miscarriage happen on its own, functioning like a bad period. I opted to come back to the hospital to get it over with.

My father dropped me off back at my apartment. He wanted to keep me company, but I insisted I wanted to be alone. I had to tell my husband and thought that should be in private. I called him and could not even finish the first sentence before I started wailing like a baby. My husband hurried home as fast as he could, jumped into bed with me and we just held on to each other. I had Gianna's parent/teacher conference scheduled for later that afternoon, but I just couldn't do it. So, my husband went in my place. He had to explain to Gianna's teacher why he was there since she was expecting me. The hospital called soon thereafter to schedule the D and C. I went the next day to have it done. I was going to be put to sleep so that I would not have to endure any of the pain, whether physical or emotional. The nurse assigned to me started very cold and almost nasty. I've always had somewhat of a young face and perhaps she thought I was a teenager. I say this because, after about ten minutes of being in the room with me, she looked at my chart and then looked at me and asked, "Oh, this is a miscarriage?" I replied, "yes, it is." She then responded with "I am so sorry. I thought this was an abortion." Her attitude quickly changed and she became so compassionate. To this day, I still feel whether pro-life or pro-choice, this nurse should have kept her personal feelings to herself and acted professionally and appropriately. By now, you know how important bedside manner is to me.

The next few weeks were emotional ones. I often found myself crying for no reason. I missed being pregnant and wanted that baby so badly. My first two pregnancies were so easy, that I could not understand how I had a miscarriage. I blamed my heart, even though I wasn't 100% sure that was the reason for losing the baby. To make matters even worse, I just reunited with my best friend after being apart for five years. She was pregnant with her first and her due date was only a few weeks earlier than mine. My husband asked me if I would be satisfied with two children, having one of each gender. They were healthy and that is all that mattered. I agreed. I put the miscarriage behind me and focused on finding us a home.

I began looking further north, approximately thirty minutes from where we were now. The town I was looking at was comparable to our current location. It fit the criteria. I found a home online that I fell in love with. It stood out from all of the rest. My husband and I went to look at it, fell in love, and made an offer.

The owners accepted our offer and we moved the following March 2007. It was a whole new world for us. I had trouble falling asleep those first few nights. The house had so many sounds that the apartment did not. I also lived on a busy street in the apartment. I was used to buses, horns, and people! Now all I heard were crickets. It took a while, but I eventually got used to it. Another issue was the stairs. My son was two and a half and I was petrified of him going up and down those steps. But luckily, he never had a fall. To this day, as I write this, I still yell at him to go up and down the stairs slowly. Of course, he never listens. But, all and all, I had a loving husband, two awesome children, and a beautiful home. Life was good.

As part of my Christmas present that year, my husband surprised me with a trip to Fort Myers, Florida. It was just for him and me – no kids. I was thrilled. We spent so much money getting the house that we stopped doing fun things and making time for one another. We were all set to go the following month in January. Just before we left, I had made an appointment to have my routine echo. It had been a while and I was due. I made an appointment with my cardiologist for a follow-up and the test results that same week. I didn't give it much thought as I was excited about Florida and busy preparing for that.

In addition to having access to the patient's medical records because I worked where I did, I also had access to my records. I stated earlier that I never used my access to look at someone's personal medical history for my gain. However, how could my history be included in that?

What was I doing, violating HIPAA on myself? I am by no means a doctor, but I like to read my findings and decipher them for myself. The report this time seemed a little different. There were words like "severe" and "intervention" that was not in all of the others.

My co-worker was good friends with one of our nurses, so I asked her to read my findings and let me know her thoughts. I was told it was no big deal and to ask my cardiologist about it. I would find out later on from my co-worker that this nurse said, "Oh, this is bad," but my co-worker did not have the heart to tell me the truth. I somehow knew something was wrong and, although I only had to wait two days to see the doctor, it felt like an eternity.

I was earlier for this appointment than I had ever been for any other. This appointment would become a changing point in my life. What I mean by that is, up until now, my heart condition was a nuisance at best, one that I did not pay much mind to other than surgery for my breasts or giving birth. However, after this appointment, I had no choice but to acknowledge the problem, and at the same time, coincidentally, my health started to decline.

The doctor explained that my bioprosthesis

had run its course. I got a good 21 years with it, but it was no time to be replaced. Somewhere over the years, I had gotten the impression that when the time had come for a replacement, the procedure wouldn't be so invasive, it wouldn't be open-heart surgery. They could just repair it through my shoulder or something. This was not the case. I needed open-heart surgery, the sooner the better. I felt like I had been stabbed right through my heart at that moment. I held back tears and swallowed hard. "Can I wait until the summer when the kids are on summer break and not in school? It would just be better on everyone involved." The doctor agreed I could wait but insisted I have it done right away if my symptoms increased. I agreed. I went back to my office, a hysterical mess. My makeup was all over the place. I was supposed to be getting excited about the trip that I was leaving for the next day, but all I could do was cry. My boss was busy reprimanding someone in her office when I came back in. She took one look at my face and told my coworker to leave her office. I explained what I had just been told. I asked to please leave for vacation right then because I could foresee myself not doing much work in the next couple of hours. She agreed.

I went home and told my husband. He consoled me and told me to only think about going away and having a good time. We would deal with my medical issue when I returned. My parents picked up the kids and I had a glass of wine. The next day we left for Florida. I had a good time on vacation but thought of the surgery constantly. There were a few times I left my husband in the hotel room and just sat on the beach, staring at the water, hoping that I would stay alive long enough to see future vacations.

I got through the next few months just by staying busy. I had two kids to take care of and a full-time job. I fainted several times, and my cardiologist told me I could be experiencing fainting spells because I was waiting so long for surgery. I met with the surgeon my cardiologist recommended. He was pretty popular and the patients spoke highly of him. I liked him and agreed on a date for the surgery. The day came and I begged my husband to take care of my kids in case anything happened to me. I thought there was a good chance I could die and wanted to make sure my kids were taken care of. I got through the surgery but as you will read in the next chapter and throughout the rest of my story, it is always an adventure, and there is always drama when I am hospitalized.

I went to the pre-op room and changed into a gown. The nurses washed me down and started an IV. They began the anesthesia moments later. I was asked my name over and over again so they could verify they had the right patient. God forbid! I woke up in recovery for a moment but then drifted right back off. In the ICU, it was the same thing. I was heavily sedated, so I slept through most of it. I remember my husband leaning over me and me saying "I love you" in sign language. I also remember the tube being down my throat. I gagged from it at one point and threw up in my mouth. Since I had the tube in, I could not spit it out, so what comes up, must go back down. I had no choice but to swallow it. Yum. I've come to hate that breathing tube and I fear that almost as much as I fear surgery itself.

After a day or two, I was moved to a regular cardiac unit where I was monitored by nurses and doctors. My co-workers provided entertainment during my hospital stay. One came to visit me during her lunch hour. Around this time, the drainage tubes were being pulled out of my stomach. My coworker opted to stay in my room while this was happening and watch it go down. I would have chosen to wait outside, but as long as I was ok with it, so was she. Gross, but whatever. My other co-worker just had no filter. The day she came to see me, a woman was visiting a patient – her mother. They were in the room next to mine. I guess she did not have a babysitter that day and brought her young child to the hospital with her. The child screamed and screamed. I was drifting in and out of sleep because of the medications. Every time this child screamed, I jumped. Well, my last jump was

75

enough for my co-worker. She jumped up from the chair she was sitting in and pushed open the door to the next room. I then heard her say, "can you shut that thing up?" She had no kids of her own. If she did, she may have thought about it first before not reacting the way that she did. She walked back into my room and sat in a chair. And I thought I was bad? I said, "Are you crazy? If I was that mother, we would be having a fistfight right now." No sooner had I said that did the mother come marching into my room, cursing and the whole nine yards. She did turn to me and apologize though. I don't remember much else after that except a few nurses coming in and stating they would both have to leave if the fighting continued. They also told the woman to not bring her child back as the hospital is no place for children.

After about a week after surgery, the doctors allowed me to give myself a sponge bath. I was so excited. Although it was a semi-private room, I had no roommate. I couldn't wait to bathe myself! I pulled the curtain around my bed and undressed. I started washing when I heard several men and one woman talking. I peeked around the curtain and the cleaning crew decided that my room would be their hang-out spot. I yelled at them to get out. One of the men replied that he was there to mop the floor. I told him if he did not leave at that moment and didn't return until my bath had well been completed, my floor would be mopped with his face. They left. I continued washing.

It was not easy returning home and stepping back into where I left off. I had no responsibilities when I was a kid and had surgery. This time I had to be a mother and a wife while I recovered. My family understood, but how do you explain to a four-year-old that you can't make him his favorite snack or you can't lift your arms high enough to brush your daughter's hair? And as far as being a wife? You try having sex after your sternum has been broken and you have to make sure your heart rate does not increase!

My mother came to stay with me for one

77

week and cleaned my house. She drove my kids back and forth to their activities. My sister came the week after. Tammy did all the cooking, so at least my husband had a clean home and meals to eat once he returned home from work. As for me, I looked like a monster but felt like a princess. My meals were prepared and brought over to me, I took naps and watched tv all day. I was waited on hand and foot by everyone around me. Except for the kids. I was still a slave.

I stayed out of work for three months. The FMLA act allowed me to do this and I was fortunate enough to have a boss that allowed me to work from home. She came by my house occasionally with work for me to do and we would chat. It was nice to stay in my pajamas and still collect a paycheck! I also focused on getting into shape once the doctor gave me the ok to work out. I went back to Weight Watchers and lost some weight. I mentioned having a breast reduction earlier. When the pounds started coming off, the first place to lose them was my chest. I went from having triple D's to barely making it into a size B cup bra. "What have I done?" I now wanted breast augmentation! Why didn't I try losing weight first before I had surgery? But the weight started to come off in other places as well, making my face look skeletal. I decided to stop watching what I ate and focused more on toning my body. I put some muscle on and my boobs grew back. After those three months flew by, I returned to work.

I was pretty much all healed by the end of the summer and back on my feet. By this time, Gianna was going to be starting middle school soon. I was worried about the earlier dismissal she would have. I would still be at work. My niece didn't care for her school and my sister was looking to move. So we decided that my niece should move in with us so the girls could go to school together and Gianna wouldn't be alone. We enrolled my niece in the middle school in town. The girls were done with school by two pm. Still, I was so afraid to have them be at home by themselves at such a young age. I told my boss I would have to resign. We agreed that I would come in each day and work most of my hours. I would then leave to go home and work the rest of the hours there. This would go on for about three years. Work-wise, it was great. I still got my paycheck but was able to get all of the kids off the bus, cook dinner on time, and spend quality time with my family. There were minimal issues. It was another mouth to feed and there was not an extra bedroom for my niece to call her own. But we handled it appropriately and made the best of it. Had I not needed surgery, I wouldn't have gotten the opportunity to work from home. When this happened with my niece, I had already proven to my boss that I was capable of working from home and could be trusted.

For that, I considered it a blessing in all of this.

Chapter 5

"Mia Isabella" (2008-2012)

As I stated earlier in the previous chapter, my niece was staying with us. She was at the age where babies fascinated her. She thought they were adorable. Since she enjoyed her childhood playing with dolls so much, a real baby would be that much more exciting. I always knew she'd grow up to be an awesome mom one day. As I write this, she has three kids and is one kick-ass mother! But back then, she was too young to have a baby. This led her to focus on me as the baby-making machine. My niece assured me that all I had to do was give birth. She would feed it, bathe it, play with it and even get up in the middle of the night with the baby! Of course, I would never agree to that. She could help out a little but that's all. I eventually got pregnant, not that we were trying to conceive. But if you take a female who is allergic to certain chemicals in rubber (condoms) and cannot take birth control pills due to a pesky heart condition, one has to try to follow the "pull out and pray" option. Have you seen the percentage of failures? So needless to say, I became pregnant once again. I was so excited to tell my niece. This was going to be better than any birthday or Christmas gift.

Once I confirmed the pregnancy with the doctor, I stopped at the drugstore to pick up "Buttpaste." For anyone who doesn't know what that is, it's a cream used to put on a baby's buttocks to help a diaper rash. I found the name amusing so I chose this product to wrap and give to my niece. Coincidentally, her birthday was approaching. We were having a family party so it was the perfect opportunity to make my announcement. My husband was the only one who knew at this point. As she opened gifts, I saved mine for last. I did buy her an actual gift but wanted the cream to be opened last. At first, she was confused. She asked me if she had a rash on her butt. Then she said, "Oh my god, are you pregnant?" I nodded and she screamed, followed by everyone else! There were tears of joy as well as concern. But my miscarriage had been a fluke thing and I did give birth to two healthy babies. What could go wrong?

After all these pregnancies, I know eight weeks was the magic number for when the obstetrician wants to start examining you and follow the pregnancy. This time was no different. I made the appointment and went. I was scheduled for a transvaginal ultrasound. The young tech proceeded to begin. As soon as she placed the probe, her face changed. She moved the probe around for a few minutes and then told me she'd be right back with the doctor. She then left the room. I started to panic. "This can't be happening again," I thought. "What will I tell everyone? What will I tell my niece? She'll be devastated." I was probably in the room by myself for a minute or two, but just like before, it seemed much longer than that. I started having bad thoughts. My dream wasn't going to come true. I always wanted three kids and when we had the miscarriage, I told myself to be grateful for what I have and forget what I don't. But now that having three was becoming a reality, or so I thought, I was excited. I did not want to be disappointed again or suffer a loss.

The tech came back into the room with my doctor right behind her. The doctor picked up the probe and began to perform her examination. After a few minutes, she put the probe down, gave me a pitying look, and began telling what I already knew. "Sorry, Stacy. This pregnancy is not viable. There's no heartbeat. These things happen sometimes. It probably was due to too many chromosomes entering the ovaries. If the pregnancy continued, it could've become an ectopic pregnancy or resulted in a baby with down syndrome. But to know for sure, we can perform a D and C and send a sample to the lab for verification. Do you think you would want to do that?" I replied with a weak "yes" and the doctor told me she would set it up. She then told me that I could try again but should wait for at least three menstrual cycles before doing to allow my uterine lining to return to normal. Both the doctor and tech then left the room and I sobbed like a baby.

It was not easy telling my family, especially my niece, but they were very supportive and concerned for me. It took some time to get over the grief, but once I did, I was gung-ho about becoming pregnant again. I was feeling a void and needed it to be fulfilled. My life had to be full, or I would just feel like that weak little girl again who could never do anything as "normal" people did. I did everything in my power to conceive.

My husband was a good sport about it. I mean, what guy wouldn't be? The website, WebMD, became my new best friend. I researched ways to become pregnant, the best times to get pregnant, and more. I even analyzed my menstrual cycle to see when my "window of opportunity" for conceiving was. My cycle has never been regular. It can be a range of between 25 to 35 days. This meant several days as being possible fertile days with only a 12-hour window.

I had to be proactive and drink lots of espresso at night! The doctor said to wait 3 months to be safe so I did. I didn't want to take any chances of having a 3rd miscarriage. By this time, I was 35 years old. This was my last chance, age-wise and health-wise. Besides, Gianna was about to be 12 years old!

Fast forward to when my 4th period was due. Well, that bi-atch just never showed up! I was excited and nervous at the same time. I spent the next four weeks telling myself to hope for the best, but expect the worst. Going to that 8th-week appointment was torture. What should have been joyous, was nerve-wracking. I also chose a different Ob-Gyn group. I was starting over (hopefully) and didn't want any bad vibes. Plus, since we had moved, I wanted a hospital closer to my house. If I was taking this pregnancy to term, I'd been told 3rd babies come fast!

I held my breath as, once again, I lay on the table, and out came the probe. "This time will be different." I thought to myself as I held my breath. Then I felt like I was in a dream. I was hearing the tech but told myself that it was too good to be true. "Congratulations, Stacy. Your baby has a strong heartbeat." I asked her if she was sure. She assured me she was and showed me the heartbeat. The tech proceeded to print several sonogram photos. She told me to wait for the doctor who will examine me but all looks great. I wanted to believe the tech but didn't want to be disappointed, so I told myself to expect the doctor to come in and tell me the tech was wrong. After a while, while just sitting there, staring at the photos in my hand, my doctor came into the room. She examined me and told me my uterus was right where it should be. She then told me to get dressed as she prescribed prenatal vitamins. She advised me to schedule another appointment for next month and gave me my due date. Out the door, I went, with the biggest smile ever. I may have even skipped a little.

The number three will forever be my good luck number. I was about to have three kids and it took me three times to conceive a third baby. I wanted to enjoy this pregnancy. Now that I was past the eighth week, I could relax a little. Again, my best friend was pregnant at the same time and due just a few weeks after me. I had a buddy whom I could talk about all things "pregnant" with. Since this would be my last pregnancy, I wanted to do all there was to do while being pregnant: maternity photoshoots, belly molds, etc. My maternity wardrobe needed refreshing, too. The first time around, I had my sister's hand-me-downs. No offense to her, but styles had changed from 1992 to 2011. I wanted to wear fitted clothes, fitted to my belly that is. I no longer had enormous breasts, so I could buy shirts to support my stomach and not so much my chest. I treated myself to A Pea in the Pod, which was an upscale maternity brand. I also had some weddings to attend, so I purchased a low-cut, long, black maternity dress. Who says pregnant women cannot be sexy. Hey, that dress made me feel that way even though I was rocking a basketball in my tummy.

My husband and I had trouble choosing a

name. Before we knew the baby's sex, we couldn't decide on either a boy's or girl's name. Even when we learned the sex, we still couldn't decide! We found out we were having a girl. With our other daughter named, "Gianna," we had to choose something that wasn't plain. Her name wouldn't be chosen until she was being pushed out.

We decided to take the kids to Disney World before it became unsafe for me to fly. Frankie had never been there and with a new baby coming, who knew how long it would be before we got another chance to go. I had always been advised not to ride rollercoasters because of my heart condition, but now I had a double whammy of being pregnant. I never listened when it came to the heart issue, but for the baby, I cheered on my family with both feet on the ground.

With my daughter, Mia, I went into labor unlike the first two. It was a nice day in August. My mother-in-law came up to pick up the kids and take them to lunch. I was spending the day with my niece and my mother. We were going shopping. Plans often change and this was one of them. While waiting for my mother to pick us up, I started getting contractions. My niece looked alarmed and said, "Should I call Mima?"(my mother). I told her to wait in case it was a false alarm. I suggested we time the contractions. Eight minutes later, I got another one. I noted the time and, again, we waited. On the dot, eight minutes later, it happened again. I looked at my niece and said, "Call Mima." My niece squealed and dialed my mother's cell phone. All I could make out from that conversation was "Mima, come quick! Aunt Stacy is in labor!" What usually is a thirty-five-minute ride from my parents' house to mine, took my mother twenty minutes this time.

My mother ran into the house, grabbed me and my bag (which had been packed for two weeks already), and put me with my niece in the car. We only made it a block before we came to a dead stop. There was construction on the main road and only one lane at a time could pass. Two teenage boys on bicycles were about to pass our car. My mother rolled down the window and yelled over to them. "Can you two nice boys ride your bikes up to the construction workers and ask them to start moving this lane, there is a woman in labor!" They said ok and sped off. The next thing I know, we were cruising. My mother honked at the men with bright yellow vests as we passed them. (laughing)

After we parked the car at the hospital (I was dropped off in the front), we went straight to my doctor's office. The nurse put me in a room right away to change into a gown and lie down on the table. The doctor came in, felt my cervix, and said, "Oh yeah, you're five centimeters dilated already. Head up to Labor and Delivery. I'll call them to say you're on your way up. I'll meet you there." She left the room and I sat there for a second, only for a second because this baby was on her way! I couldn't believe this was happening. My dream was finally happening. After all the heartache and disappointment, here I was. I got dressed, met my mother and niece in the waiting room, and said, "Let's go! We're having a baby!"

Once I got to the L and D floor, the nurses greeted me and whisked me away to a room. I changed into a robe, got into the bed, and was hooked up to many machines. My husband got there about an hour later, followed by my mother-in-law and my two kids. She said, "I just left you!" My father joined us soon thereafter. Once it came time to start pushing, my husband and mother stayed along with my daughter and niece. My niece would have filmed it if she could! Everyone else waited outside. Four hours later, my Mia Isabella was born. During the final pushes, I pleaded with my husband to settle on a name. I don't believe anyone should be born nameless. Everyone is someone. We agreed on Mia as the name. And Mia was perfect! She came out with hair, all ten fingers, and toes. Frankie and Gianna could not stop staring at their new sister. My niece couldn't wait to hold her. Later that day, after everyone left, I was left alone with my new baby. I whispered, "I can't believe you're here." My life was complete.

Fast forward to going back home and getting settled. If I thought having two kids was a lot, welcome to three! I had a middle schooler, a kindergartener, and a newborn. Holy moly! When two were content, one needed something. There was never a dull moment. Mia was breastfed, so she got up every two and a half hours to nurse. You would be amazed at how many great shows are on tv between 2 and 3 am!

My new daily routine was so busy that I started to feel sluggish and exhausted. I returned to work after three months and we had a full-time babysitter to take care of Mia while I was at work. I stopped producing milk when Mia was about two and a half months, so I no longer breastfed. Yet, I still didn't feel right. I shrugged it off as post-pregnancy symptoms and that my body was returning to pre-pregnancy so my hormones were out of whack.

I attended my friend's son's birthday party. I told my friend about the symptoms I was having and how I felt. She had recently given birth too, so she assured me it was just a post-pregnancy thing. Then abnormal symptoms started happening. Things that I never did before. I would get this urge to stretch my body over and over again for about a minute. My hands would become itchy and I would rub them like crazy until the feeling went away. Then there were the chills. It was warm out, yet I would get a chill that would last about a minute or so. My body would shake so much that my neck would hurt. Then as if I snapped my fingers, it would stop. I made an appointment to see the doctor. I saw the physician assistant who told me I had had some sort of virus and left it at that. I was told if the symptoms continued, to come back. So, I went home and didn't think much of it.

My symptoms continued, however, and they seemed to be getting worse. I made an appointment to see my cardiologist since I was due anyhow. He suggested drawing blood cultures on me to see if that told us what the deal was. Anyone who doesn't know what a blood culture is a blood test on both arms. The sample is then evaluated for about five days to see if there is a growth of bacteria in your bloodstream. So, I did that test. I also made another appointment to see my general practitioner. Since her PA told me to return if the symptoms persisted, and I did so. This time I saw the doctor. She also wanted to do blood cultures. I explained that they were just done. Since both doctors belonged to the same group, there was no need to repeat the test. I would just have to wait. So, I went home again. The next day I went to work as normal. After work, I got back in my car. The temperature read 90 degrees, which was extremely warm for April, yet, I was freezing. I drove home with the heat on full blast. I knew then that something was very wrong. I got home and the babysitter greeted me. She glared at me "You don't look well. I'm calling your mother." I just wanted to lay on the couch and rest. The next thing I knew, both my mother and father were at my house. My mother took my temperature and told me it was high. I started having chills again,

95

shaking all over. My mother became nervous. "That's it, we are going to the hospital," I begged her to stay put, but again, this is my mother we're talking about.

Chapter 6

(2012) "Some Smart, Some Dumb"

We drove to the local hospital and I was checked out by the doctor on call in the E.R. Again, I was told I had a virus and to follow up with my doctor. So, I went back home with nothing accomplished... again. I resumed my routine of going to work, still feeling like crap. Upon arriving home, I barely made it through the door. I was shaking so much and burning up. My babysitter put me in her car and she said we are going to the hospital. I asked her to take me to the one by my parent's house. She agreed since the one near me did squat. She called my mother on the way. We all got to the hospital at the same time. My husband was meeting my babysitter to grab the kids and drop them off at my sister-in-law's house. He wanted to get to the hospital to be with me.

The hospital was baffled by the symptoms I had and why I had a fever. They had no idea what was causing this reaction, so they admitted me to run several tests. The next day, the blood culture results came back with a positive result of having bacteria in my bloodstream. I was scheduled for a TEE echocardiogram. Normally, I have a TTE echo, but since this was a little more serious, I needed this type of test. A patient is put to sleep so a small tube can be applied down the throat. I woke from the procedure with a sore throat, which I was told is normal. The results would come back in a few hours. The doctors told me that I most likely will need strong antibiotics to tackle this bacteria and it can be done at home. I was relieved. I had a life to get back to. I had a husband and kids who needed me. But why couldn't the other hospital figure this out? The doctor came in with the echo results a few hours later and told me the dreaded news. "Stacy, you have very large vegetation on your prosthetic valve, also known as bacterial endocarditis. We have to operate to remove it. If it breaks off and enters your bloodstream, it can be life-threatening." I felt the wind get knocked out of me. "This can't be happening. Am I in a bad dream?" The doctor continued. "Your cardiologist wants you transferred to the hospital in the city. They are more equipped and prepared to handle this type of situation. You will be transferred by this afternoon. This can't wait. We are sorry," The doctor walked out, I looked at my parents in disbelief and started to wail like a baby. My parents squeezed my hand and told me it would be ok. They would be right by my side the whole time.

The hospital I was in arranged for me to travel to the other hospital via ambulance. I had an IV pole, so traveling any other way would be impossible. The ride was about a half-hour. My mother was allowed to ride with me. I just kept staring out the back windows thinking what if another car slams into us and I die, not from heart failure, but from a car wreck – wouldn't that be some shit! Once I arrived, the hospital staff quickly whisked me away to the cardiac floor.

They put me in a room that already had one occupant. There was a bathroom in the room and it smelled like urine. At the time, I didn't know if it was the bathroom or my roommate that smelled. (laughing) I would eventually realize it was the bathroom! My mother tried to make it better by putting a soap with a cucumber & green tea scent in it to freshen it up. To this day, I cannot use that soap. It smells like human pee to me. The same goes for what I use for the litter box. I don't clean anything else with it. It reminds me of cat pee!

Up until this point in my life, I rolled with the punches; meaning, I did everything I was told by the doctors, never questioned anything, and accepted it all. I had had enough. When I tell you the nurses, the doctors poked me so many times with needles, it's an understatement. I was not a happy camper. To make matters worse, my soon-to-be surgeon walked into the room. He introduced himself first and then things got serious. He told me the surgery could not wait, I was scheduled for the next day. "Already?" I asked. I was told what the other hospital said previously and then some. Because the vegetation was so large (broccoli size) if it breaks off and enters my bloodstream, I will go into cardiac arrest within minutes. I could die. He continued speaking. "I am a pediatric surgeon but am experienced and competent to perform surgery on adults. This is an emergency and cannot wait, so the hospital needs to use who is available. Don't worry." He then left and I cried again. Now with this new news, I became angry. I never felt sorry for myself, but now I was questioning it all. My mother tried cheering me up, but there was nothing she or anyone could say to make it better.

Still feeling pissed off an hour later, a phlebotomist walks in. She proceeded to tell me that she had to do blood cultures on me. "For what?" I said, followed by my mother who asked the same question and then some. "We've already established that there is a growth and she is scheduled for surgery tomorrow. What could this test possibly reveal in five days that we don't

101

already know? Is this necessary? Her arms are sore and beat up from all the needles." This chick replies that she is just following orders. So, we agreed to it and asked her to please be gentle as my arm was bruised. I barely got a nod as a response. She irritated me so much that I clenched my fist not for the blood draw, but with the desire to punch her. She started to put the needle in my arm and I said "ow." She lifted the needle and placed it in another spot. I said "ow" again. The next moment, I will never forget. I think I lost all control of myself because I turned into an exorcist. She lifted the needle, put both of her hands in the air, and said, "Baby girl, I didn't even touch you yet." Blood at that point began to trickle down my arm coincidentally. I looked at her and said, "Then why is my fucking arm bleeding then?" She argued something to which I cannot recall, I just remember my mother telling her that she stuck me because I was bleeding. I stood up in bed, pulling all the wires I was hooked up to, and started yelling. "Get the fuck out of my room, you incompetent bitch!" My heart monitor skyrocketed and my mother pleaded with me to calm down and lie back down. My nurse, followed by other nurses, ran into my room. I told them to get her out of my room and she is not to return. If they need my blood, they will have to send someone else. The nurse assigned to me, whom I did like, drew my blood without incident. I apologized to my roommate who told me not to worry about her, she just felt bad for me. She was entertained. I would have several more uncontrollable seizures' that night, registering in the 160s heart rate on the monitor.

The next morning started with the usual surgery prep. My body was washed and sterilized. I could have nothing to eat or drink. Every Tom, Dick, and Harry came into my room that morning – they were the assistants to the surgeon, who was the anesthesiologist in charge of watching my blood pressure and heart rate. I just wanted to start and get this whole ordeal over with. If I made it through this time, I had a family I had to get back to.

Finally, the time had come. An orderly came to bring me down to the O.R. My parents followed. My mother held my hand the entire time. I was brought into the surgery prep room.

They put me onto a gurney and put warm blankets on me. My husband was meeting us there. He worked for a little bit to tie up loose ends so that he could take some time off to be with me in the hospital and at home. The time was nearing the surgery and I began to get nervous. "Where is my husband?" I needed to see him, maybe for the last time, and have him assure me the kids would be taken care of. He called my mother and I was told he was circling the hospital. There was no parking anywhere! My older niece volunteered to drive his car around to look for parking so he could see me. Little did I know, I would be there for another two hours.

The Physician Assistant walked over to us and told us that my latest MRI revealed a small mass on my brain. As if I needed anything else wrong with me. They had to have a neurologist look at it and examine me before I could be cleared for surgery. "Great." I thought. "If my heart doesn't kill me, my brain will." We ended up waiting two hours for the neurologist to come. My surgeon and his assistant put on music and began dancing and drinking coffee. Had I not been so nervous, I might have laughed. I was worried that my surgeon would become tired and not perform his duties well. (laughing). I expressed this to them. The staff assured me that these things happen all the time and not to stress over it. Just when I was about to lose it, a man who I can only describe as Bleeker from the Muppets, walked over to me with his entourage of medical students. He explained why he was there and what he was going to do. When I tell you that his exam could be performed by a five-year-old, I am not joking. He snapped his fingers in my right ear to see if I could hear it, then did the same thing on my left side. Then he asked me to follow his finger as he moved it in front of my face. He took a step back and said, "She's all clear.

Proceed with the surgery." My surgeon and his staff yelled "Woohoo!" As for my family and

I, we looked at each other and said, "That's it? That's what we waited two hours for?" My surgeon walked over to us, told me to get the show on the road, put a surgical cap on my head, and released the brakes on my gurney. I waved and blew kisses at my family as I rode off. Once they were out of sight, tears rolled down my cheeks.

I know enough now to know the surgery protocol. You are rolled into an extremely cold room. It takes about three people to hold onto the sheet you are lying on top of, lift you and slide you from the gurney to the O.R. table. Once there, they start hooking you up to all kinds of machines. The area of your body being operated on is wiped down and iodine marks the spot. Lastly, a mask pumping anesthesia is placed over your nose and mouth. They then ask you to count backward. In all my surgeries and being put under, I don't think I ever counted past 97.

I woke up in Intensive Care the next day. A breathing tube had been placed down my throat.

Remember I said I hate those? 2008 came to mind. The whole gagging on it and being forced to swallow my vomit because I could not spit it out. This time, I began to choke. I banged on my bed rails to get the nurses' attention. I could see them in the distance. To this day, I am not sure what they said, but I believe it was: "Let's get this out of her, she's crazy." Had I not been too weak in the chest, I might have verified what they said and then proceeded to tell them off.

A morphine dispenser had been placed next to my bed for pain. I was allowed to press it every ten minutes. No one else had authority. One of the nurses from the tube incident walked over to my bed to ask me how I was feeling and then told me that I should try not to press the morphine button if I could handle the pain. I nodded, but when she walked away, I mumbled, "Right, ok, you dumb bitch. You feel what I am feeling and tell me that you would TRY not to press it?" I spent the next few days in the ICU and then was transferred to a "Step Down" unit. I probably could write a book based on that experience alone! (laughing).

I wanted the window side but it was already occupied by an elderly lady who looked like she'd been there a while. The room had a nice view of the river, but it was of no benefit to me since my roommate did not offer to open the curtain that separated us. The husband came daily, bringing many things from their home. It consisted of blankets mostly. Nevertheless, there were times that they cooked. Yes, I said cooked. Sometimes my room smelled like fish. The nurses often had a hard time getting to the patient because of all the crap around her bed.

There was a day when I was scheduled for an echo. The technician came to my bedside along with the portable echo machine. I couldn't be moved yet since I was hooked up to a lot of machines. The technician drew the curtains around me. If anyone knows anything about an echo, you are naked from the waist up, so the machine gives a good view of the heart and its chambers. The husband of the patient sharing the room with me peeked into my curtain and asked what test I was having. I'd find out later he was a doctor back in his country. But he startled me and I quickly raised the bed sheet to my chin. The tech said, "Excuse me!" and quickly closed the curtain. She then yelled at him to mind his own business. She apologized to me and continued with the test.

Sponge baths were a daily thing for me as I had a catheter in and was attached to other machines. They assigned a male nurse to me one day. I refused to undress or show any parts of my body to him. I told the head nurse to do whatever she had to do, but I wanted a female nurse. They made the switch. The male nurse looked annoyed, maybe because he thought he was getting a chance to see a body other than an older man or woman, but to him, I would say, "Not today, dude; at least not with me."

They finally removed the catheter because it annoyed me so much. They tried using bedpans with me. I don't know about you, but they don't work for me. I cannot relieve myself lying down. Plus the thought of missing and getting any on my sheets is just gross. I am no bed wetter! One simply does not pee in bed. I don't eat in bed either. That's freaking gross. The nurses finally agreed to no more bedpans, but I would have to ring for my nurse if I had to go. I was still hooked up to the machines and a little off balance. I agreed. As long as I could pee in the toilet, so be it. I wasn't concerned about the other stuff. Medications often constipate me, so I knew there would be a while for that event.

The next day, I had to pee badly. I rang for the nurse – no answer and no one came to my room. I rang again. Still nothing. I started disconnecting myself from the heart monitor and other machines. My IV pole had wheels, so that wasn't a problem. The bathroom was only a few feet away so I could make it. What I didn't know is that I was connected to two machines under my bed. They drained the fluid out of my body daily. As I began to walk to the bathroom, these machines fell over, spilling all the liquid inside. I

110

started shouting and my nurse heard that one! She came running in, asking me what happened and why I got out of bed myself. I replied, "Well you didn't answer and when you gotta go, you gotta go." So, I got a chance to pee and my floor was cleaned. I apologized for being a nuisance, but I still felt they should have been more attentive to my needs. Being here was hard enough.

So, as if this wasn't already enough drama for me on the Cardiac floor, the time came to change my sheets. By this time, I was allowed to take an actual shower. I just couldn't use a razor since I was on blood thinners. If you have ever seen a hospital towel, you know they are not that big. I wrapped myself in one after my shower. It barely covered my ass. However, my bed was three feet from the bathroom, so I didn't mind much. I closed all the curtains around me and started to change. I suddenly heard a woman's voice telling me through the curtain that she needs to change my sheets. I replied, "Just a minute, I'm changing." She then tells me she is on a schedule and repeated that she has to change the sheets. I repeated myself. She repeated herself for the third time. At this point, I wrapped the towel around my waist, (I now have a top on) and rip open the curtain, I tell her, "I said I am changing. You can either wait a minute for me to finish changing or I will gladly pee on my sheets first – since I'm not wearing pants yet – before handing them to you, you inconsiderate bitch." She left and filed a complaint about what a rude patient I am. Oh well.

Breakfast was the highlight of my day in the hospital – except for visitors of course. The lunches and dinners, not so much. Dinner was served at about five o'clock each day. At home, I eat dinner around the same time but often munch on snacks thereafter until I go to bed. So at nine o'clock one night, I was starving and bored. I at least wanted a snack to munch on while watching a show. I begged my father to buy me some snacks. He left and came back empty-handed. "I'm sorry Stacy, the cafeteria is closed." Visiting hours had just ended so my parents packed up to leave. I kissed them goodbye and sulked. Not even five minutes later after they left, a cart rolled by in the hallway filled with snacks.

But! Nothing for me, because you see, I had no money on me. "Why the hell would I need money in the hospital?" The very next day I would have my father hunt the cart down and buy some snacks before he left for the night. And my bed tray drawer had a stack of one-dollar bills.

I woke up one morning to the Physician's Assistant staring at me, nose to nose. He was a bit of a jokester and to be honest, probably kept me from losing my mind during my hospital stay. Anyway, he told me that the latest x-ray showed a lot of fluid around my heart and it needed to be drained. It wasn't urgent so he waited for me to wake up. He knew I had been having a hard time sleeping here at night. The draining of the fluid is a simple process, one that can be done at my bedside and with me being awake. The only thing was, I had to be very still. He would be the one to do it, along with the head nurse whom I liked. I agreed that is until he whipped out this ten-inch syringe with a long-ass needle. "What the hell is that?" I shouted. "I've seen knives with shorter tips than that!" I cried. Tom, the PA, told me it was not as bad as it looks. He offered me a washcloth to bite down on. I told him that he couldn't be serious and no freaking way was that needle coming anywhere near me. He told me I didn't have a choice. The fluid would continue to build up, causing many complications health-wise. So, I reluctantly agreed. Tom reminded me to remain still, but as soon as the needle started approaching, I began to fidget. Tom turned to Sharonda, the nurse, and told her this isn't going to work. "We may have to knock her out." "Knock me out?" I asked. "Yes, please." He replied, I'm gonna punch you and, then you'll be knocked out." I couldn't help but laugh. I said he was a jokester. (As I write this, we are Facebook friends.) They gave me anesthesia right there in my room and off to sleep I went. I woke up a little while later alone in my room. Tom came to see me a little while after and told me the procedure was a success. I had a bandage and the site would be sore for a while, much like getting a flu shot. It would leave a permanent one-inch horizontal scar below my right armpit. I sighed. "What's one more scar?" I can now play Connect the Dots on my body.

A few days before being discharged, the doctor came in to talk. He told me that he had gone over my medical records with colleagues and, although the vegetation was removed, they wanted to ensure there were no more bacteria in my system and also wanted to prevent any other growth from happening. To do this, I had to be put on heavy-duty antibiotics through IV. My choices were to spend the next six weeks in the hospital while the staff administered the medication or to go home with a PICC line and administer it myself. My jaw dropped when he said six weeks. So, the latter was the obvious choice. "What is a PICC line?" He explained that it was like an IV tube that would be taped to my arm and the medication would be administered through it each day. I could shower but not get the site wet. If I chose to go ahead with it, I would undergo a small procedure to have it inserted in my arm. I would be awake, but the only pain I would feel is the initial pinch much like a shot.

I weighed my options: spend six more weeks here or go home in a day or two. It was still long-sleeve weather, so no one would see it on my arm. I chose the PICC line. I did not want to spend six more weeks here. I would go crazy! I told the doctor my decision and he made arrangements for the procedure. The good news was the daily blood draws can come directly from the PICC line. I would no longer be stuck with a needle.

The next day, two nurses, older than the norm from the ones that I had daily, came to see me.

They told me that they are PICC line nurses and would be the ones doing the procedure later that day, in my room! I said, "Uh, are you sure that's sterile?" They chuckled and said it was, there won't be any incision larger than a regular IV. I signed some paperwork and they told me they'd be back.

Later on in the evening, the nurses came back. This time they had loads of equipment. The whole side of my room turned out looking look like an O.R. There were machines and sterile disposable mats everywhere. My entire body was covered, except for my right arm. One of the nurses began looking at my veins on a screen while she ran a doppler over my arm. I told them that I didn't have very good veins – it takes a lot to get my blood. "Nurses often tell me I have rolling veins. One second they're there and then they disappear." The two nurses laughed. "Did I miss the joke?" I thought. One of the nurses said, "Oh, these young nurses… When will they learn? Veins DO NOT roll!" They found my vein after a minute or so, gave me a pinch, and started working the tube through my arm. All in all, it wasn't bad. Catheterizations are worse. I just felt a little queasy from seeing some of my blood on the mats. The whole procedure took about forty minutes and the tube outside my arm was about 10 inches. The nurse looped it around and held it together with a bandage. She showed me how to do it when the time came for me to change the dressing and off the nurses went. After that, for each staff member that came for a blood sample, I gladly showed them my PICC so as not to get jabbed!

My surgeon visited me after that to see how I was doing. He asked me if anyone had explained how this happened in the first place. I shook my head "no." He told me it was something foreign that landed on my skin and made its way internally. They don't know what it was and I may never find out. From the beginning of all this, I was asked numerous times if I had been to the dentist. Dental work that increases blood flow, is a major possibility to result in endocarditis. I always have to be premedicated before having any dental work. This time, however, I hadn't had a visit to the dentist recently, so that scenario was ruled out.

To elaborate more on the whole dental thing in regards to bacteria, my risk of possible exposure ensured that I probably will not get to accomplish something I wanted to do before I grew older and began losing my teeth. I was born with an underbite, meaning my lower jaw sticks out further than my upper jaw. This results in what I think is a terrible smile. I also have extremely small lips. So, smiling even without showing teeth does not look nice on me. I often pose for photos with a "duck face." Not because I want to look sexy, but to not look butt ugly in pictures. I would love to have corrective surgery to have my jaw realigned the right way and smile nice. I don't care about the pain involved. I've now had three open-heart surgeries and brain surgery. There isn't much more that's more painful. I am a happy person and smiling is just something that I wish came easy for me. But because of the risk of bacteria and infection, it's not a wise thing for me to pursue. People often suggest that my pose of the "duck face" is to appear sexy, especially when viewing a photo of me on social media. That's why I decided to mention it. My lips don't look like that. I am happily married and in my forties. I am not trying to attract the attention of the opposite sex or get "likes" or "followers" on my page. If I could smile nicely, I would, especially for photos with my family.

Anyway, the surgeon began to question me. "Any tattoos?" "No." "Body piercings?" "No." "What about manicures and pedicures?" "Of course." "It is unlikely, however." He mentioned. I couldn't help but smirk. "Great, cuz I'd be dead by now if that was the case." These were just some of the things they mentioned could be from. I would spend the next year, afraid to cut myself shaving (hence buying the expensive razors), get a Mani/Pedi, drink from the office water cooler, etc. I often found myself running to my bathroom at home because I refused to even step into a public one. To this day, I still avoid public bathrooms whenever possible, even if I have to hold them in for hours. But I've always been that way. Public bathrooms just gross me out. And forget the bathrooms at the beach! You are probably in flip flops, so your feet are exposed to the ground. How do we know that the ground is wet from people coming from out of the ocean and not because they peed on the floor? Eww.

The day before I was discharged, I was presented with several companies to order antibiotics from. First things first: do they accept my insurance? Once I made my choice, I was told a representative from that company would pay me a visit to sign the paperwork and explain how the process worked. An Infectious Disease doctor came to see me. She explained that she would be monitoring my medication and how I was progressing. I needed to have my blood drawn weekly to look for any signs of bacteria. The PICC line could be used for that and the draws could be done at my general practitioner's office. While she was going over everything, the representative from the medication company walked in. Together, they explained how it would work, when and what comes daily, the times to administer it, etc. The doctor told me that it was very important that if I see any bubbles in the tube working its way down into my arm, I am to "flick" the tube to break the bubble. Air in the line was not a good thing and could be harmful. Ok, not much scares me, but that did. I had confidence in the nurses, but myself doing it? Not so much. The first few times I watched the nurses as they administered the medication, closely paying attention to how they removed the air bubbles. The following day I was discharged. I signed all the necessary paperwork and hugged those that left a positive impact on my stays like Tom, Sharonda, and several nurses. I told them as much as I wanna see them again, I hope I don't, at least not in this setting. Off I went, in a wheelchair that is.

After spending eight days in the hospital, I was home – or should I say my mother's home. I now had an IV pole and medication that came daily on ice. My mother wanted me to stay at her house so she could monitor me. She wanted to make sure the antibiotics were being administered correctly. The air bubbles scared her as well. That first night in her house, I needed a dose of antibiotics soon after leaving the hospital. The company I was ordering the medication from, already had sent the first delivery as promised. My sister, together with her boyfriend, hooked up the IV pole. They started to give me the medication. I warned them about the air bubbles. Paul, my sister's boyfriend, now my brother-in-law, said "Oh yeah, watch out for those." He is a former EMT. I told them what the hospital said about it is crucial to get air bubbles out of the line. Paul told me it wasn't that serious and that I wouldn't die. He and my sister were laughing and I think they enjoyed flicking the bubbles. (laughing)

My mother had set the spare bedroom up for me, IV pole and all. She forced me to turn in early, telling me I needed my rest. "What am I five?" She had to wake me at 2 am for another dose, and again at 6 am. It was like feeding a newborn and I was the newborn! So, like a good daughter, I listened and went to my room and watched tv. I had always been a person who slept on my stomach. With the PICC line, I had no choice but to lay on my back to sleep. I eventually fell asleep and as promised, my mother came in at 2 to give me my dose. She stayed up until it dripped through – about twenty minutes or so – then disconnected the PICC from the IV tube. She went back to bed and I saw her again at six. She looked exhausted. I told her to go back to bed, I could manage to disconnect myself.

She argued and I argued that she had to be fresh and polished for me later that day. She reluctantly agreed, eventually, and went back to bed. I must have fallen asleep because the next thing I knew it was after seven and my IV line was filled with blood. I started freaking out, yelling. I thought that I would be sucked dry if I was disconnected soon. In reality, I have lost more blood from a razor cut from shaving than this. My parents came running in and disconnected me. They assured me I was ok, but my mother blamed herself for allowing me to do it myself. I felt bad. I also felt like a failure since I

124

told her I could handle it but I didn't. Later that day, we returned to my house, even though my mother fought me on it. After the fiasco we just had, my mother wanted me to stay at her house for a few days so there would be no distractions and she could continue to monitor me, but I missed my husband and kids. My hubby had been holding down the fort in my absence and was doing a phenomenal job, but I needed to be home. My mother gave in but I couldn't get rid of her that easily. She packed her bags to stay at my house. Not that I wanted to get rid of her because I did not; I was calmer and more confident in my healing when she was around. I felt safe.

Once we got to my house, my mother made me go right to the couch and sit. She told the kids that they were allowed to kiss me only. Hugging might hurt me, let alone jumping on me. They were not to, under any circumstances, bring any drama or issues to me. If they fought, she'd kill them. She hovered over me like I was royalty. My mother took off for work, just like she did in 2008, and was spending the first week back with me at my house. I couldn't bend over and get worn out easily. I took a nap each day, mid-afternoon. My mother cleaned my house daily, cooked, and tended to the kids in my place. I didn't even have to get off the couch. She brought my meals right to me. By the end of the week, I'd say she needed a vacation! Around this time, a rash started developing around the area of my PICC line and also on my other arm where several IVs had been placed. The rash progressed quickly and started to become painful. Ice was the only thing helping. I couldn't take any over-the-counter medications like Benadryl since it could interfere with my antibiotics. Ice worked while I was awake, but how could I keep it on when I went to sleep? One night it became so unbearable, that I thought I would rip my skin off. I got up, took a pair of my husband's old socks, and cut both ends off. I then filled two snack-size Ziploc bags with ice. I slid a sock up each arm and placed an ice bag between my skin and the sock. I did fall asleep and it got me through most of the night until I woke up soaked since the ice had melted. From all the bandages on my arms through the years, I must have developed a latex allergy, and this time would become the first of several allergic reactions to it.

My sister came the following week, again just like in 2008, and like my mother, she also took a week's vacation from her job to take care of me. She made many meals for us and tended to the kids. I woke from a late nap one day to her burning a side dish. She was running around the kitchen sweating. I asked what the hell was happening. She told me the baby had taken a huge crap and she had to change her. She wanted to wash her down before she put a fresh diaper on her. That was great and all, except she, forgot she was frying some tostones on the stove at the time. Well, I learned what burnt plantain tastes like that night. All in all, I enjoyed my mother and sister staying with me. I am truly grateful and we shared many laughs. Especially when my sister put on plastic gloves and a mask to give me my meds, but the mask kept rising, covering up her eyes. Little did we know it would be practice for

Covid. It took ten minutes just to send the antibiotic through because she couldn't see! I had the PICC line pulled out of my arm several weeks later, completing the course of antibiotics. All in all, it wasn't bad. I just had one incident where my son had an event at school. A mother that I was friendly with, saw me, came up to me, and hugged me. I had a long sleeve sweater on so she had no idea. She squeezed my arm so tight, that the Picc line pinched me. I thought I'd faint from the pain. I stars.

I'd like to say the rest of that year was uneventful, but it was not. I was hospitalized two more times before the year was done. The first time I went back after the bacterial infection was because the PICC line had gotten clogged and my medicine could no longer flow through it. I had to go back into the hospital for around-the-clock antibiotics to prevent infection and had to have a new PICC line inserted. Only a few weeks later, I returned to the hospital once again. This time with viral pneumonia. And boy! This one tested me mentally!

During my inpatient stays, I had a total of six different roommates two. Each got to come and go while I stayed. They were always older. Some were coherent, some were not. The second night I was there from my PICC line problem, I had a woman assigned to my room named Jane. Jane had lost her husband a few years ago and her daughter was in charge of her care. The daughter left for the evening once Jane was settled in. She never opened her curtain but I heard the tv, so I just put mine on and left her alone. Some time between 2 and 3 am, I was awakened by whimpering. I opened my eyes but the room was dark, so it took me a few moments to adjust to the light. Once I could see clearly, I saw Jane hovering over the large garbage bin situated between our two beds. I could see her IV wire stretching from the pole over to her wrist. She was saying, "help me, help me. I am trying to pee." I yelled, "Hold on" and pushed the nurse's call bell quickly. When they answered, I told them my roommate needs immediate attention and that they need to come quick before she falls.

Moments later, a few nurses rushed in. Lights switched on everywhere. They helped Jane back to bed and my nurse thanked me for calling them. The lights go off. The next morning, Jane walked over to my side and apologized. "I had to go badly. At home, I have a commode by my bed. I was confused and couldn't understand how it got so much higher." I tried not to laugh. It was funny, but I felt bad for Jane. "It's ok. I get it."

As if that wasn't enough drama, this time I went back in for a pneumonia infection. Only this time it was viral. Bacteria is a little more serious. Nonetheless, I had to be admitted. There was a patient on the floor that suffered from dementia. Every day and every night, she would scream at the nurses. She would yell that they were hurting her. She accused the doctors of trying to kill her and any staff member that was a male, she accused them of trying to rape her. It was brutal to listen to. I prayed to God that I would be discharged. Both visits were a week each. At least the food was decent.

Chapter 7

(2013-2014) Game Changer

By the beginning of 2013, my life had returned to its normal routine. I went back to work, and the kids went to the daycare/after-school program. I figured the worst was behind me and now I could focus on my future. Being home, and recuperating, left me with gaining a few pounds and having no muscle. I still couldn't do much in the way of lifting anything heavy, so weight training was out. But I could at least try to lose weight. I enrolled in Weight Watchers for the second time, but this time I was doing it solely online. My old job had started a program once for WW. My friend and I joined as I was getting married at the time and wanted to lose some weight. Well, she and I were the laughingstock of the group. All the women in it had fifty or more pounds to lose. We wanted to lose twenty or so and become healthier. Plus, being in our 30's when everyone else was in the late forties–early fifties did not help the situation. It quickly became toxic and my friend and I eventually stopped the program. The women were cruel and somewhat bullying. The nerve of them! These women probably needed the program more than me and would probably kill to be my weight, but that didn't give them the right to shame us or feel guilty for being the way we were. Don't get me wrong, overweight individuals should never be teased, bullied, or ridiculed because of their size. I feel sorry for anyone subjected to this type of behavior. But no one has the right to shame someone else for wanting to better themselves, skinny, heavy, etc.

So I did WW online. It worked for me! I combined this with daily lunchtime walks around my place of employment. In three months, I had lost 20 pounds and increased my endurance. I could walk up hills without being winded. That was something I never felt before. It felt fantastic. I felt normal. My cardiologist noticed too and commended me.

For the next year, I continued to maintain my new weight loss and continued walking. Once I became totally healed from surgery, I began lifting weights. Nothing crazy, just enough to tone. Life was good. I had a job, a husband with 3 awesome kids, and a beautiful home. What more could I ask for?

Forty was quickly approaching, but I didn't think much of it. Life was normal. I ran to work every day, sent kids to school, came home after work, made dinner, did laundry, and helped the kids with their homework – the usual shit of an average working mom. Life as I knew it, was pretty routine. The only change happening was my family convincing me to get rid of my cherry four-door Jeep. It was approaching eighty thousand miles and started having mechanical issues. I loved that vehicle. It kept me young. I felt like a badass in it. And at the same time, I could fit all the kids in it with their hockey bags and take off. Now, I was losing it. My Mia was still young and I was told a Wrangler was not the best vehicle for a baby. There are too many bumps and such that come from driving it. So in the end, I traded my beloved "Tank" for a Honda Pilot. It was nowhere near my Jeep, but it had so much room, including a third row. It was a great vehicle for a hockey mom!

For my birthday, my husband gave me a trip to Punta Cana, Dominican Republic. I was ecstatic, to say the least! If that wasn't enough, we were staying at the Hard Rock. I heard stories from people that went there. They all had the best time. I was super excited. After all, I could show off this new body! For the next few weeks, I watched what I ate, bought new outfits, and planned an itinerary for us. My mother and father were graciously watching the kids the whole week for us. The day before we were leaving for D.R., I got a mani/Pedi. We ended up having a blast on vacation. I would return the following year and the year after that, but things would never be the same.

We had just gotten back from vacation and Christmas was around the corner. I was running around like crazy. I had to shop for gifts. I promised the kids we'd make cookies and I needed an outfit for my company's office party. I kept getting headaches but just shrugged them off because I was always on the go and never relaxing until I fell asleep in my bed. Finally, I saw the doctor who sent me for an MRI. At this point, I still wasn't thinking much of it. I had several things on my mind to stay busy. Then a few days after the test, my coworker asked me if I wanted to go somewhere for lunch. She also had been doing a lot of running around and just wanted a change of scenery. We went to the local pizzeria/trattoria for lunch. I don't think I will ever forget what I had for lunch that day. I will explain why later on. When our lunch was over we walked outside and saw that it had begun to snow. It was just enough snow to be beautiful and the perfect accent to this time of year. Upon arriving back at the office, my friend went ahead of me as I stopped at my car to get something.

Afterward, I walked inside the building and over to my suite. I bent my head down to shake out the snow that had fallen in my hair and onto my coat. I felt a "pop" in my head, followed by a throbbing pain. I walked into the office. I turned to walk to the right, but my body kept walking straight. I knew something bad had just happened to me.

I managed to get to my desk, slumped into my chair, and threw my head back. My co-worker started talking to me. I told her I didn't feel well and what had just happened. A couple of other coworkers came rushing over. One of them brought me aspirin and water. They told me to just sit. I tried getting a hold of my cardiologist to see if he had any pull with getting my MRI report. I wanted him to look at it, even though it was a brain scan. I thought maybe he could interpret it and give some insight into what just happened. He was out of the office, though. The staff didn't know for how long. I tried again a little while later but got the same response. I decided to email my boss. She was out also and wanted to let her know I was leaving early. I just didn't feel right and work was the last place I wanted to be. So, I packed up and left.

On the way home, I decided to stop at the mall and see if I could find an outfit for my company holiday party. I had some time before I had to pick up the kids and since time was usually non-existent in my world, I went for it. I walked into a store, looked around, and saw a top that caught my eye. I asked the sales lady if they carried it in my size. She told me to check on the table underneath for different sizes. I bent down and that same "pop" went off again. I knew I had to get out of the store and to a doctor. I somehow managed to get to my car, but I was walking sideways even though my brain was saying to go straight. I fell against my car, pushing the button on the key fob to open the door. After several attempts, I got the door open and crawled in. I could feel my face drooping. I took a "selfie" to see what I looked like. It looked like me, but only much more miserable and my face appeared to be lopsided. I did the next thing I could think of, I called my mother.

For the next thirty minutes, I sat in my car, in the mall parking lot, talking to my mother on the phone. She pleaded with me to let her call an ambulance, but I refused. I knew they would just take me to the hospital that was ten minutes away. The same one that misdiagnosed me two years earlier with the bacteria. My mother hung up and then called me back a minute later. She had gotten a hold of my husband and he was on his way to get me. He called his sister who was picking up our kids for us from their daycare and hanging on to them for the time being while we figured out what was going on with me. So, I continued to sit there, in my car, watching the sun go down. I told my mother I was going to hang up because I wanted to rest. At first, she said no, but I told her I would hang up anyhow, so she said goodbye, that she loved me and that my husband would be there soon – to hang on.

My husband pulled up along the side of my car. He opened my door and pulled me out and put me in his car. I looked at him as though I was being rescued by my knight in shining armor, a moment I'll never forget. I told him to take me to another hospital and not to the one I mentioned earlier. The next hospital was about twenty minutes away.

On the way there, I felt the right side of my face fall more, including my lips. I squeezed my husband's hand and cried, "I don't want to die." My speech was slurred as I said it, alarming me even more. My husband squeezed my hand back and told me that I wasn't going to die – he wouldn't let me, he loved me very much. We pulled up to the E.R. Steve jumped out and ran around the other side of the car to get me out. My parents were already there, standing on the curb along with a nurse holding onto a wheelchair. I fell into my husband's arms as I was getting out of the car. I couldn't stand up. "Why not?" I thought and panicked. They all sat me in the wheelchair and rolled me inside. The next thing I knew, I was on a table with about six people, nurses and doctors combined, hooking me up to all kinds of machines. None of them knew what was happening to me. I threw up all over myself.

The doctors were baffled by the contents of my vomit. They couldn't explain what looked like little stones. As much as I was far from having a good moment, I chuckled to myself. They were staring at pieces of mushrooms. I had a chicken marsala pizza for lunch. I ended up being admitted to the hospital so they could run tests. The following morning a lady came in with some applesauce. She asked me to swallow some. She gave me a tiny bit. I couldn't! I freaked out. She explained that whatever was happening, I lost the ability to swallow. It could be temporary or take longer. "What the hell is wrong with me? Who can't swallow?" I also developed pneumonia, just as I did in 2012. Only this time it was worse and I needed a Bipap machine to help me breathe. I also couldn't see anything with this monstrosity on my face. I could hear my family in the room talking, but I couldn't see them. I think the doctors gave me heavy sedatives due to my discomfort because the next few days following this is a blur. I just knew something bad had happened, and I couldn't swallow. Once the doctors had exhausted all possibilities of a diagnosis, they wanted to perform a spinal tap. My mother got very upset and claimed the hospital did not know what they were doing. She got on the phone with the hospital coordinator from my job. Soon thereafter, I was transferred back to the city, to the hospital that healed me in 2012.

Once I got to the hospital in the city, I bypassed the thousands of people in the hospital lobby. I was taken to the Cardiac Care Unit and greeted by the best nurse (We're Facebook friends too!). She quickly stripped me down and changed me into a hospital gown. She told me she was doing it quickly to not come across as aggressive, but to get it done before any males walked in and to avoid me being embarrassed. As luck would have it, my monthly friend decided to visit me. Barno, my nurse, was very professional and discreetly handled it. I had known this nurse for five minutes and in the many, many experiences I've had with medical staff, she is by far the best and also my favorite to this day. We met again after this whole ordeal, but that's for another chapter.

An echo TEE was scheduled right away. The doctors wanted to make sure bacteria did not reoccur and were causing this – something this hospital was already doing that the other hospital didn't. The test would be performed right in my Cardiac Care room. A team of six nurses and doctors filled the room. As I stated earlier, the patient is put to sleep for this exam. I woke up a little while later to find myself alone in the room. I panicked. It took me a second to realize where I was. I felt groggy. It was like something out of a horror movie, where a victim wakes up from being knocked unconscious and tied to a bed in an unfamiliar setting. I rang for the nurse. Barno came rushing in and assured me all was fine. She explained that there was no telling when I'd wake up, so the staff left with the notion that she would stay on alert for when I woke. To this day, however, I still feel it was unprofessional of the staff to have me wake up with no one in the room, even though my nurse came right away. What if

I didn't know to call the nurse or couldn't find the call button? They knew I'd be confused. The echo TEE was interpreted soon thereafter and showed no signs of any bacteria. That ruled out the cause of what this was. I was relieved since that was so tough to experience, but so was this. It was scary – what was happening to me. I wanted answers.

That night, around one, am, (late, no?) I was scheduled for an MRI. I had one in the previous hospital, but this current hospital wanted its results. This test would be the one to answer all the questions and give me a diagnosis. So, I went to the basement of the hospital to take the test. The orderly wheeled me into the hallway and left me there. He explained that the technician would be out in a minute to get me. He then left. I was alone again. The hallway was dimly lit. Here we go with creepy again. I was just waiting for Michael Myers or Freddie Kruger to attack me. After about five minutes, or what felt like five minutes, I was about to hop off the gurney and see what was up. Just then the technician came out of a door, greeted me, and wheeled me into the room she had just come out of. The MRI took about an hour. The tech wheeled me back into the hallway and told me the orderly was page. He would be here soon. She then disappeared. "Here I go again." I thought as I laid there. But by this time, I was too tired to care. It was after two in the morning and I had had a long day. I shut my eyes. The orderly appeared a few moments later. I crawled into bed upon getting back to my room. At least I could walk.

The following morning, a cardiologist that I was familiar with since he was a doctor from the group I worked for as well as a colleague of my cardiologist, came to see me. He was the doctor assigned to see the patients that were admitted to the hospital. He explained that the results had come back from the MRI I had the night before. "I have some good news and some bad news," he said. "The good news is we know what caused all of this. The bad news is..." I braced myself. I was thinking of either a heart attack or cancer. "You had a stroke, Stacy." "What? Isn't that for old people?" I asked. He said it could happen to anyone, but there has to be an underlying issue somewhere. A blood clot traveled from my heart to my brain and I had a stroke. "So, my heart did this?" I was confused. I knew I had a heart defect, but I didn't think I was at risk for anything. The doctor told me it wasn't necessarily my heart. "What about the mass they found on my brain?" I asked. "It's possible. Your last echo revealed no abnormalities with your heart, so I don't believe it caused the stroke." I was then told that I may never know what did it, just like I don't know what gave me bacteria. "I am a walking, breathing, time bomb, waiting to explode." I thought to myself. I'd live in a bubble, but even that won't stop any malfunctions within my body. "I'm sorry," he said. I had to fight to hold the tears back. "Ok, so what happens now?" I asked. "Will I never be able to swallow again?" The stroke also caused right-sided weakness and temperature was non-existent on that side as well. He placed his hand on my shoulder. "Time will tell all, Stacy. Everything could come back tomorrow, or you may never be the way you were." I took a deep breath. "I have one last question, please." He nodded. "Why couldn't the other hospital tell me this? I had an MRI there as well. " He stared right into my eyes. "Sometimes a stroke can take a few days to show up on the test. It never came out on the first MRI." I must have looked dumbfounded. I still wasn't satisfied. "I had all the symptoms of a stroke. Anyone can search for a stroke on the internet and read about the signs. This should absolutely be the first thing that comes to the mind of the doctors. I could have been spared from the effects had they done something right away. How horrible! There are no words." Now I let the tears roll. He looked sympathetic at this point. I could tell he felt bad for me. "This hospital wanted to be thorough, so they repeated it because that's what we do. We can't undo what they did or didn't do, but we can certainly do everything to try to get you better. You're in good hands now. Have faith." The doctor then left my room and I cried and cried.

The first few days really sucked. The stroke

caused hypoxemia, so I needed oxygen treatments several times daily. I also had total numbness on one whole side of my body. I couldn't feel anything on my right, so it was kind of a blessing when a blood sample was needed. I didn't feel the pinch from that or when the IV had to be changed. I had a really sweet nurse named Catherine. She offered to brush my hair, and do other nice things to make me comfortable and relaxed. Sometimes I'd catch her staring at me. Almost like how a person stares at someone they adore or idolize. I would ask her politely what she was thinking. "Oh, nothing." She would then hurry out of my room. One evening my older niece came to see me along with her girlfriend. Yes, she is gay, lesbian, homosexual, or whatever word you go by. Hopefully, it's a respectful term at that. She is one of the most loving genuine people I am blessed to have in my world. Anyhow, they walked into my room. Catherine was there taking my vitals. I introduced them to one another and Catherine left me to be with my visitors. When Catherine was out of earshot, my niece, Raeann, spoke. "That one is definitely gay." Her girlfriend, Vanessa, laughed and my jaw dropped. "No way!" My niece rolled her eyes at me. "You don't think I know my own people?" I laughed and said, "Well, that explains it all!" I told them about the care and stares. "Yup! The nurse is sweet on Aunt Stizzle." Vanessa chuckled. I just rolled my eyes. But I did feel a little funny every time Catherine came by after that. Not because she was gay, but because I am married. Regardless, Catherine could have been a hot guy and I'd still feel the same!

The days continued and swallowing food remained unsuccessful, but I was hopeful that at any moment, I could do it with ease. I was scheduled for a barium swallow x-ray later that day. I was looking forward to it. Although the saline in the IV kept me from feeling hungry, I wanted to eat and taste real food. My nurse (not Catherine) came in later on and told my mother and me that the test had been canceled by the doctors with no explanation. My mother rose from her seat and began yelling at the nurse. "She has been looking forward to this all day. What if she can swallow now and you're holding food from her for no reason?" The nurse told my mother she would speak to the doctors and left the room. My mother looked at me and said, "I'm sorry. They don't know their ass from their elbow." The nurse came back a little while later and told us my test was back on. I caught my mother wink at me.

If you never had a barium swallow test, it goes like this: you are brought to an x-ray room, and they sit you down and cover you with a protective mat to protect you from radiation. At first, you are given a few sips of water to swallow while a team of doctors together with technicians watches a video and studies images at the back of your mouth, throat, and esophagus to see how you handle swallowing. They look to see if the water flows down your esophagus or pools in your throat. I managed to swallow the water with no problem. Next, the technician handed me a spoon of applesauce. I tried to swallow that, but to my surprise, I couldn't. The doctor told me to swallow hard, and I did but felt the applesauce in my throat. I started coughing. The doctor said there was no need to go on. He said he cannot allow solid foods at this time since I could choke. I was devastated. Other than not having the ability to eat, mealtime was the only enjoyable thing on a hospital day besides visitors. My mother tried to cheer me up. She told me at least I'll probably lose weight. That was true, but I was too sad to care at that point. Swallowing is normal and should come naturally. I couldn't swallow therefore I wasn't normal. Why didn't anyone understand that?

That test would be repeated two more times before I left the hospital. I failed both times. There were no changes. The doctor told me I could only stay on a saline drip for one more day. I had to get nutrients in me or there would be other problems. I held out for one more day, hoping my swallowing would come back. But I was starving and felt weak. A nurse, whom I wasn't crazy about due to her bedside manner – or lack of, told me I would have to have a tube inserted through my nostril to the back of my throat to pass nutrients through. She told me I wouldn't taste the shake and the tube won't hurt being inserted. She proved herself to be full of shit. To this day, I'd like to say incompetent also. She began to push the tube up my nostril. Well, it hurt like hell. Imagine a cotton swab going up there, only wider, longer, and harder. She just kept pushing. I heard my nose crunching. I yelled for her to stop and she told me she wasn't doing anything to harm my nasal cavity. However, my nose started to bleed. I'd say she harmed it somewhat, asshole. To this day, when I sneeze, it is about 5 or 6 sneezes at once. My family waits until I stop to say "Bless you." The next day, the tube slipped out of my nose, resulting in me tasting the shake. I think vomit tastes better. The tube was taped to the space between my nose and lips to hold it in place. It blocked part of my vision. It came right off. The nurse tried taping it again. It lasted a half hour. I went back to drinking a lot of water and starving.

The next morning, a gastroenterologist came

to see me. She told me about a procedure they can do to give me nutrients and it didn't involve a tube up my nose but through my stomach. I didn't know whether to be excited or nervous. The doctor puts you to sleep and then makes a small incision in my stomach and puts a feeding tube in. That would mean I would get my nutrition from special cans designed essentially for this. These cans were like protein shakes, only they also contained some fat and carbs. With the feeding tube, I definitely would not taste the shake. At this point, Christmas was a couple of days away. I wanted to be home more than anything, especially to be with my family.

Nutrition was the last piece of the puzzle. It was determining whether or not I could be discharged. I did not care at that point if I had a hole in my stomach. I told the doctor to schedule the procedure and get it going. The doctor hesitated and told me to consider waiting since it is surgery and my ability to swallow solids could come back at any time. I politely told her that I know myself and my body well enough to know that this isn't going to come right back. I prayed and did everything I could to bring it back. It wasn't from lack of trying. This was the only thing keeping me here and, if it meant going home, then we do it. She agreed, had me sign the paperwork, and told me she'd be back with the information about when the test will be. I crossed my fingers and said a little prayer. With any luck, I may just be home for Christmas.

The doctor came back a little while later and told me the date and time of the test. It was scheduled for the next day, late morning. I had two days before Christmas. The next morning, I was prepped as usual, and down I went for the test. I was told the whole thing would be done in less than an hour. I asked how long after I could go home and the doctor replied, "We'll see how you do. There will be a foreign object in your system now. Your body may reject it and it could cause complications." Blah, blah blah. If I can have valves from pigs and cows in my body with no issues, what is a plastic tube gonna do? Later on, I was brought back to my room. I was sore from the incision but had no other problems. A nurse came in to check on me and my family asked about being discharged. She said she'd get the doctor. The gastroenterologist came in and she explained that for me to go home, they have to be confident that I will be able to get the daily amount of nutrition I need. Someone will have to help me and administer it properly. Because I still had no feeling in my hand, I wouldn't be able to hold the can and tube to give it to myself properly. My younger niece, Arianna (the baby lover) spoke up and said, "If someone can teach me, I'll do it. I can stay at her house with her and give it to her on schedule." I don't think I have ever loved Ari more than I did at this moment. What 17 year old is willing to give up their winter recess to feed their aunt like a baby, but not in a cute way? She told me that she wants me home for Christmas and hugged me. My father, the doctor, and I all looked at her with amazement and admiration. The doctor agreed to it and told my niece to pay attention as she gives me my first dose of tube feeding. Three hours later, the same process was repeated.

All was going well that day until early evening. I started burning up and throwing up. The nurse and doctor came in and explained that it was my body getting used to the liquid. I had nothing in my stomach for 2 weeks and now I was filling it up, so my body was out of whack. It was nothing harmful, but I'd have to stay another day in the hospital for observation. I was devastated. This now meant I would be discharged after Christmas. I ended up going home the day after Christmas. But as I write this six years later, my life would never be the same.

Chapter 8

(2015-2016) La Phlegm

    The daily routine for my home hadn't changed much in my absence. With the help of our families, my husband managed to hold down the fort. The kids were fed, groomed, and the laundry is done and he somehow managed to keep their homework and studying in check. I slowly began to adjust to being at home and caring for my family and house. I just had to think of new ways to do things as the stroke impaired a few parts of my body. My older two children took the school bus daily. It picked them up right in front of the house. It picked them up and dropped them off, so their transportation was not an issue. I was not allowed to drive for two months. Mia, on the other hand, was in pre-k and her school was on the side of town. That was a problem. My husband had to leave for work before they even opened. I could not care for her at home just yet nor did I want her to regress if I kept her at home and then she returned to school once I could take her. I didn't know what to do. Then, it was as if God had answered my prayer. I was sent an angel. It's been said that people come into your life for a reason. I believe that. Mia's school's director had an assistant. This woman happened to be my neighbor a few houses away from me. She graciously offered to take Mia to and from school at no charge. MaryAnn even went as far as to put the car seat from my car into her car and leave it there for the duration. She continued to take Mia even after I could drive but was still home, just so I wouldn't have to make the trip. Who does that? An angel that's who. A godsend is what MaryAnn is. We are still neighbors and friends. I will always be grateful to this lady. As I write this, today is her birthday. Happy birthday MaryAnn!

As for me, I continued to have issues from the stroke. For one thing, it left me with a cough reflex. I would cough constantly bringing up phlegm each time. I'd go through a box of tissues in one sitting. My daughter, who was a young teenager at the time, gave me the nickname "La Phlegm" on her phone. (laughing) It was gross, however. I got so embarrassed if someone was around. Then, there was food. I caught several family members sneaking away to shove a piece of food in their mouths. They felt bad eating in front of me. I couldn't blame them. I'd probably do the same thing. I just felt sorry for myself. Especially through the holidays. Here everyone was enjoying a big feast, eating, and drinking, while I had my stupid cans for my tube. And that tube! I have handles on every cabinet in my kitchen, they are perfectly aligned with my belly button. I believe they are designed just so that they can grab and pull onto your tube as you try to move away from the cabinet. Talk about pain! I almost yanked it out entirely once. It was enough pain to throw up. I couldn't get it wet, so I had to bandage myself up each day before I showered. Forget taking a bath. And I'm sure it wasn't attractive looking to my husband.

While talking to my friend that came to visit, she told me that she read somewhere that a person can receive Botox injections to improve their swallowing. I looked it up online, and there was such a thing performed by an otolaryngologist. I researched specialists and found one not too far from the house. I made an appointment for later that week, praying this would be a solution to my problem. I met with the doctor at a local hospital, one that I had never been to before. I had new high hopes. This otolaryngologist took a few X-rays, reviewed my medical history, and assured me that he could help. "It is a simple procedure. I perform the procedure here in my office. But with your medical history, I think it's best if we do it in the hospital." I left his office that day feeling hopeful. The procedure was scheduled for the following week, but to me, it was an eternity. The phone at the house rang the night before I was scheduled to go to the hospital. It was someone from the otolaryngologist's office. I heard what they were saying on the phone but I felt like I was in a bad dream. "We are very sorry, but due to the severity of your medical history, we feel this hospital is not equipped to handle a situation if there are any complications. Your safety is our priority." I started to cry. My father grabbed the phone. Luckily, I was spending the night at my parent's house since they were driving me in the morning. My father was yelling at them asking them why wasn't this addressed in the first place and how unprofessional it is to call a patient the night before and cancel on them. They apologized and suggested contacting a physician that was affiliated with one of the city hospitals. Even though I didn't agree with how this hospital handled this situation, however, I agreed with their decision and concern for me. I respected them for acknowledging that they are not equipped enough to have a patient such as myself and to suggest that I am in better hands with an NYC facility.

So, I started over right away. Again, I researched specialists, only this time I used a different zip code. I found one that had many positive reviews in all the areas that were important to me, expertise, training, bedside manner, etc. I called the next morning and got an appointment for the following week. As these days went by, my swallowing did improve somewhat on its own, however. I could manage small bites of soft foods like ice cream and smashed fruits. It was like baby food! I still wanted to be normal, nevertheless. I wanted to eat out at a restaurant, eat normal adult food and not have a choking fit from it. I wanted this tube out of my body! Then there was my younger daughter's first birthday party to which she had been invited. It was for a friend in her preschool class. My mother offered to drive since the whole thing may be too much for me yet. My daughter was shy and would not attend the party without me. My mother offered to sit in the car for an hour and a half during the party. I still couldn't drive and had been advised to not be left alone yet, especially outside the home. I brought my daughter into the room where the party was being held. All the kids were sitting at a table while several mothers stood behind their kids. I panicked thinking I did not have enough strength to stand on my feet for that long. But I was doing this for my daughter. I missed out on so much already. I'll hold out for as long as I can. I probably would have lasted the duration of the party except where I was standing was between the back of my daughter's chair and another little girl's. This little girl was in Mia's class and obnoxious on any given day, and so was her mother. There's some truth to the apple that doesn't fall from the tree! Anyway, this little girl could not sit still. She was constantly moving around in her chair, causing the back of it to push into my stomach. It kept on rubbing up against my tube, which pinched my skin each time. I thought I'd puke.

Why didn't I move? There was nowhere to go and besides, if I moved from that spot, Mia would freak out and cause a scene. Luckily by the time, I could no longer stand it, it had been an hour. The cake was already served. Mia was

163

starting to fidget herself, so I told her we had to go. I politely excused us and told the hostess we had another party to attend and thank her for having us. I then bolted. My mother asked me why we left the party early and I told her the whole story. Being a mom, she said, "See? I knew this would be too much for you." We went home.

The day finally came for my appointment with the new otolaryngologist. I crossed my fingers and said a prayer. As they say, hope for the best but expect the worst. My father was driving me and coming along for moral support. I met the doctor and instantly felt confident in him. He had a warm, calming presence about him but seemed incredibly intelligent. He took X-rays, reviewed my history, and told me that it was a wise decision on the other otolaryngologist's part not to feel comfortable doing the procedure. After all that, he explained that this could be done, like the previous doctor, he also does this procedure in his office, but for me, he would do it in the hospital as an outpatient in case there are any complications from it. He eased my mind by telling me that, unlike the other hospital, the hospital he is affiliated with is well prepared to handle any situation that may arise from this. It did help that it was the same hospital where I had my first open-heart surgery and gave birth. I had total faith here. He gave me a date two weeks in the future. But I persisted. Ok, I begged to say how badly I needed this and wanted it, so he made it for a week later. I left, smiling, and feeling like the wheels-were finally starting to turn.

As luck would have it, (no pun intended) my procedure date was scheduled on St. Patrick's Day. I needed some luck from the Irish that day! I got up extra early, did my hair, and put on makeup. I even wore a green sweater to acknowledge the day. When I arrived at the hospital ambulatory wing, I was immediately impressed. They put me in a room with mahogany drawers for my clothes and a key to lock it. I was given a gown, unlike any other hospital gown I had ever seen. This one was disposable and covered my whole body! Have you ever worn a hospital gown for anything? They do come in different sizes but if you're a petite woman stuck with a man's gown, chances are your boobs are exposed because the short sleeves of the gown are huge. You are not safe if you raise your arms! Just don't do it!

Besides, big or small, they all suck when it comes to hiding your derrière. Crack kills. Anyway, these gowns called Bair Paws were made by the company 3M. It made a not so pleasant moment, a little more pleasant since the robe-ish gown was a little less hospital-like, even though I was grateful to be having the procedure. I was brought into a sterile room and put to sleep.

I woke up in recovery, a little groggy. A nurse was sitting in a chair beside my bed. At least I wasn't alone this time. My father was there already. The nurse explained that the procedure went well but it would take a bit for my right vocal cord to expand to meet my left vocal cord and swallow properly. This would be something they tested before I was able to go home. The procedure proved to be efficient and off I went. I was to repeat the procedure every three months as needed.

After this, I began eating everything in sight. My weight started to increase. My face became fuller. I began to unfollow my protein shake schedule and ate more solid foods orally. I had a follow-up visit with my gastroenterologist a few weeks later. She said she would remove the feeding tube if I put on at least five pounds. My father chuckled. "She did. Just look at her!" (laughing) Thanks, Dad. I stepped on the scale and I managed to put on twenty pounds since being discharged from the hospital. The doctor said, "Yes, she no longer needs the feeding tube. Lie down on the table for me." She lifted my shirt to expose my stomach. She placed a towel under my belly button. I was told to take a deep breath. The tube was then pulled out of me. It hurt like hell, but I felt free. The doctor put a bandage over the area where the tube was and told me I would be sore there for a while and would have a small scar. Other than that, I'd be ok. My first thought was that I would finally be able to soak in a bubble bath, with some music and a glass of wine. And those damn kitchen cabinets of mine! They no longer would grab me! Unless I wore drawstring pants of course!

Now that the tube was over and done with, I could address the next medical issue on the list, the mass in my head. My family asked around and was told about a highly recommended neurologist that only dealt with this thing in my brain. Another advantage was he was affiliated with the hospital that helped me recover after the stroke.

After my consultation, I was scheduled for another MRI. This doctor wanted images from his machine and if repeat images were necessary, it had to be the same machine to accurately measure any changes in growth. It was like using a scale for weight. You want to use the same scale to keep track of your weight loss. We all know the ones in the doctor's office add a few pounds to the ones you use at home!

Luckily for me, the radiology department was located only a few floors down from the doctor's office. I had my scan and the results would be sent to the doctor right away. Back to the office, I went. After examining the images and reading the report, I learned that the mass on my brain was an acoustic neuroma. It is a non-cancerous tumor that developed in my inner ear. It wasn't life-threatening but can be a nuisance. Ya think?-I had a serious thought as the doctor was telling us about this tumor.

"Can it cause a stroke?"

"Probably not. These tumors are slow-growing and don't cause any permanent damage. That said, it needs to be removed. It can affect your hearing and balance." I just always assumed I was a little deaf from all the loud music over the years. I'm married to a former DJ! Plus, I always say I'm dizzy and a klutz! I didn't like that he said "Probably not." We all know anything is possible. Especially when it comes to me!

The neurologist told me my tumor was larger than most but I was still a candidate for Gamma Knife treatment. Gamma Knife is a non-invasive, procedure that treats brain lesions with gamma radiation. Its goal is to cease tumor growth while preserving neurologic function in the brain. It would be done in the hospital as an outpatient.

My first reaction was to say, "Explain the knife." Once he told me that there was no actual knife, I calmed down a little. It was short-lived, however. He then said a frame would be placed over my head and held together with pins to hold it in place. "How is it held into place? Do the pins get screwed to my face?" I started to freak out. This doctor is extremely professional and knows his stuff, he takes his patients seriously, but I did manage to make him chuckle a little. "There's no pain Stacy, I promise." He scheduled the procedure in his book.

Here I go again with another procedure, I thought. *Will all this ever end? Or will I see at least one doctor from every specialist to treat some part of my body that is screwed up? How did I manage to have three beautiful kids with no issues? Thank God at least something went in my favor.*

The procedure was scheduled for the following week at the crack of dawn. I remember driving to the hospital in the dark. I couldn't have anything to eat or drink. That sucked because I really could have used a cup of coffee. I was brought into the pre-op room. I went through the usual, changed into a hospital gown, had an IV inserted in case I needed medication for anything, and was advised of the risks. The nurse handed me a sedative. I would not be put to sleep for this but the sedative would keep me calm. It would ease my comfort for any anxiety about the procedure itself and if I experience any discomfort from the pins touching my skin. I swallowed the sedative and sat back in the chair. It would take some time to kick in. After about forty minutes, I told the nurse I didn't feel any different. I had a high tolerance for things like Percocets, Vicodin, etc. from all the stuff given to me through the years. She gave me another sedative to take. Another forty minutes went by. The nurse came back to see me and I told her nothing had changed. She told me she couldn't give me anymore.

"You were given the same amount we give to six-foot, 250 lb men," she exclaimed.

I shrugged my shoulders and said to myself, "How much worse can it be than having a catheterization?"

I guess the sedative took its time to work, because the next thing I knew, I woke up with this thing around my head in a dimly lit room. I heard someone say, "Don't worry Stacy. You're fine. We are doing the Gamma Knife now. You passed out from the sedative. We are almost done. Try not to move." I fell right back to sleep.

Later, I woke up in the recovery room with my doctor there. He told me to see him to follow up with him after some time to see if the procedure worked and if my tumor shrunk. My head was wrapped in what I can only describe as a turban made of ACE bandages. It was heavy and I couldn't raise my head as easily as I normally did, but whatever. I survived yet another picking and probing of my personal property, also known as my body.

My follow-up was approaching and I was eager to see if the tumor had shrunk. I was nervous every day now. I convinced myself that it was the tumor that caused the stroke and as long as it remained on my brain, I was at risk for another one. I did another MRI so the neurologist could compare the first image with this latest one. I headed up to his office afterward. After some time, we finally were brought into his office. The doctor looked at me and told me he had good news and bad news. The good news was the tumor had not grown any since first being diagnosed. The bad news was it had not shrunk either. I felt the tears sting my eyes. He told my husband and me that he had done hundreds of Gamma Knife surgeries and only five had not worked. I was his sixth. Lucky me! Another procedure that I had to endure was not a success.

"So now what?" I asked as I fought back tears.

"Well," he said, "We have several surgical options, however, I would advise doing a translabyrinthine approach. It's what we do for larger tumors. It lowers the risk of dysphagia which can cause complications with Stacy's heart. The other approach is less invasive, but it is recommended for smaller tumors and has a higher chance of dysphagia."

⸗ "Ok, I have no choice. Why would I do the latter?" I questioned.

The doctor looked at me and I was shocked at his answer. "Because there is a downside to the first approach that is definite. Whereas the second approach has a chance that it will not occur. What I am trying to say is that both surgeries will remove the tumor but the first approach will leave you with no hearing in your right ear. The second approach has a chance to preserve it. But I spoke with your cardiologist and we feel with your heart condition, it's just too risky to do the second method."

My husband then asked the doctor if I would have any hearing left. The surgeon pulled out a wall phone from his desk and pulled the cord out of the receiver.

"She will be like this." I swallowed hard and my husband gasped and looked shocked. I guess the doctor could read our faces because he then spoke.

"I know this comes as a shock. But it is not as bad as it seems. You may not even notice you can't hear in that ear unless you're wearing headphones or switching a phone from one ear to the next. You may just have some trouble hearing someone over any other noise in the background. I did the same surgery on an 18-year-old girl. Like you, she was scared. I followed up with her recently and she told me the hearing loss has not affected her and she lives her life normally. This won't affect your speech either as you may notice

175

in some people with total deafness."

I had one more question. "Will you have to shave my head? Having long hair is important to me. Any hair for that matter. One bald person in a relationship is enough." (laughing)

This is nowhere near the severity of anything happening to me medically and you may be questioning my priorities but as I said, it is important to me. It was hard enough with scars all over my body and a crooked smile. Plus, one puffy foot. The doctor told me that they shave a small spot and that I have so much hair that it would probably not even be noticeable. I guess my facial expression said it all because he continued speaking. "Look, think it over. I know it's a lot to process. I don't need an answer now. Call me with any questions or concerns. One thing is for sure however, it has to come out." With that, I shook his hand, and out we went. I cried all the way home.

Even though the doctor said it was a lot to think about, there wasn't. I had a top-notch surgeon with a top-notch hospital. He was a colleague of my cardiologist so they'd be working on this together for my benefit. Unless I cut my head open and tore the tumor out myself, I had to do this. I just had to get past feeling sorry for myself and work out the timing. After all, I had a job, kids, that depended on me, and more. I called the surgeon's office the next day and scheduled the surgery.

Chapter 9

(2016) Do you hear what I hear?

By now, from reading this you know the drill as well as I do. I went to the hospital, was taken to the pre-op room and had to remove my clothes and put on a gown. I had to remove my nose piercing. I tried taking off my wedding rings, but they would not budge. I hadn't taken them off in years. I've just cleaned them while wearing them. Of course, I wasn't the same weight as I was in my twenties, so my fingers got fatter. The nurse tried taking them off but failed. I told her she only succeeded in making my finger swollen. It may have been a rude remark but with me, you get what you give, and she was rude from the beginning. So fuck her. She told me if I can't get them off, they will have to be cut. "No way," I said. "I will call off this surgery before that happens and lose weight. I don't care about the materialistic part of it. but the rings themselves mean a lot to me. Family is what has gotten me through all of this. I can't destroy them." The nurse continued her spiel on how important it was to have this surgery and how risky it is to have any type of jewelry on. You are probably thinking *Where are your priorities?* and I should be thinking of the bigger picture. If there was a way around this, I was finding it. The anesthesiologist came over to get some medical history on me. As soon as he introduced himself, my nurse proceeded to tell him about my rings. I think even before he finished introducing himself. It was almost like we were children and had a fight so she tattletales on me. The doctor looks at my hand, says it's no big deal, tells the nurse to just cover it with medical tape, and asks me if he can ask me some questions. Of course, I agreed but not before rolling my eyes at the nurse.

I woke up in recovery hours later. The right side of my head hurt like hell. The nurse in the room told me not to touch my head. But as soon as she walked away, I did just that. It felt like a bunch of staples from the top of my head down to my ear. I still could hear everything around me so for a brief moment, I thought my hearing was not affected. I knew that wasn't the case as soon as someone came on my right side and started speaking. I could hear them speak but not loud enough to make out what they were saying. I also saw the bottom of my hair hanging down my face, so they gave me some relief.

ICU is like the presidential suite of hotels but for hospitals. I had my room with my butler. Ok, nurse. You don't get out of bed for anything. They bathe you, bring your meals and come as soon as you ring for them. The only downside to this is that because they stay close to you, they are right outside your door, so in the middle of the night when you are trying to sleep, they're busy chatting away with co-workers. Their voices keep you up. I once asked the nurse politely to keep it down. The second time she woke me up by talking, I told her to shut up! She pleaded with me not to report her.

"I don't snitch," I replied. "I just want to sleep. Being here is hard enough to rest without you being a chiacchierona." I don't know if she understood that word but heh, she was acting like one and I like to say it!

The day came when I no longer needed to be in the ICU. I was being moved to a Step-Down unit on the neurological floor. All I had ever known was the cardiac and maternity floors. So, this would be an adventure. Boy, was it, and not for the better! My IV had gone bad so the ICU nurse told me that they were going to change it before moving me. They were more experienced in ICU than in the Step-Down unit and wanted it to be more pleasant for me. Well, it turned out to be a disaster. I might have puked or even fainted had I not been through so much of this already. The nurse could not find a vein anywhere.

She checked both of my arms numerous times, sticking me each time. The needle would go in but she couldn't push a syringe through. The nurse ended up calling a vein specialist who came with a little machine. He told me he could see where my veins were on the machine. Well, that was a big fail also because he had to move the probe around on my arm to look for veins and once he found one, struck me, and tried to push the syringe through, but it would not work. Both arms were bleeding. The blood was starting to drip on my sheets. I was hurting, my heart was racing and I was sweating. It took a total of one hour for them to give me a new IV. One hour! Did I mention that the IV was now in my foot? Never, ever, and I've had numerous IVs, have I ever had one in my foot!

Right after they moved me. It was late. I had no family with me. They had already gone home. My feeling of happiness in finally getting through that fiasco was short-lived. The room in the Step-Down unit I was put in had three other occupants. I have never stayed in a room with more than one other roommate. It was like a scene in a horror movie. One where the psych ward is the setting. There were four beds in the room, each with curtains drawn around them.

The occupants consisted of two males and one female. Males! What the hell? I didn't even think that was allowed! Remember what I said about being in the ICU back in 1987? That moment came rushing back to me. I hated everything about my new quarters. The nurse assigned to me looked like she hadn't brushed her nappy hair in weeks. She had so much hair on the side of her head, I don't know how she held her head up. When she bent over me, her hair touched me. I got so skeeved out, I'd thought I'd vomit right there. Then the lady next to me had a breathing machine. She sounded like she had been a smoker all her life. I vowed right then and there to never pick up another cigarette ever! She just sounded horrible, manly, and gross. The man across from me was no better. Every time he hacked, he sounded like a monster. Someone used a bedpan at some point and the room began to smell. That was enough for me. I called my husband and told him that if he does not come to get me, I will pull the wires and tubes out myself and will walk home. I meant it too. He said he would talk to my mother who was staying at my house to help my husband with the kids. I refused all medical attention including medication, meals, etc.

Look, I am not better than anyone, nor do I consider myself a diva or high maintenance, but this was ridiculous. I was not a drug user or hurt myself intentionally. I have real internal medical issues and deserve to be treated well. These conditions were unacceptable. I let every staff member know too. I was not staying quiet.

I guess I made such a fuss because at 3 am, the nurse practitioner came into my room, shining his flashlight on my face. This guy was six feet tall, with a high-pitched voice. Anyway, this dude shines the light in my face and says, "Honey, what's the problem? Your mother is calling here over and over, demanding that we move you, or she is calling the local Congresswoman."

"First, you're not my husband, family member, or friend. Don't you dare call me

"Honey" "Secondly, it would be in your best interest to get that light out of my face!" He left.

My daughter then sent me a text to ask if everything was alright. From her bedroom downstairs at home, she could hear her grandmother, my mother, on the phone, screaming at the hospital staff about me. My husband also sent me a text to say my mother was losing her mind on them. I was moved to a private room that morning. Thanks, Mommy.

My new room had a nice view of the river and the bridge. I also had my private bathroom. Put up some picture frames and a fresh coat of paint, this could have been a basic hotel room. Once I got settled, the nurse assigned to that wing came to see me. She told me that I wouldn't see her as much as I normally see my assigned nurse. This wing is just for observation so while the care is there, it is minimal.

"That's fine," I said. "I just need medication, and an occasional look at the incision, no?" It turns out my stay lasted longer than the norm. I developed viral pneumonia....again. The doctor suggested I caught it during surgery from having an open wound. I suggested I caught it from that disgusting room they first put me in. Even with pneumonia, they just had to give me an antibiotic. It was detected early enough so no other intervention would be required. As far as my brain was concerned, as I mentioned above, the doctors and nurses just checked the surgical site for signs of infection and to make sure it was healing correctly. *I could be at home for this*, I thought.

The next day was my father's birthday but he was spending it with me at the hospital to keep me company. My mother was taking him out to eat that night. They both needed a break. While sitting there talking, a head nurse walks in to tell me she has to move me since they have a patient coming in that had to be quarantined and because I developed pneumonia. ─I should be moved further down the hall for better observation.

"Are any of the other rooms semi-private and not have four together?" I asked her. She replied, "No, they're not."

"Well, then I'm not moving."

"The patient who needs this room has an underlying condition and cannot be compromised." the nurse told me as if that would have made a difference.

I became agitated. I too have an underlying condition, a heart condition. I've already caught a staph infection once. I do not intend to risk having another one. I think it's best if you look elsewhere. Besides, a nurse can't walk another ten feet to my room to check on me? Really? She left and my father left saying he'd be right back. He came back a few minutes later with a patient handbook. "Read this," he told me. "Know your rights." The nurse came back again and brought a friend. I laughed at her. Did she think she could intimidate me with her backup? So this nurse didn't smile. So what? No longer was I. The fact that she just tried to bully me, pissed me off even more.

My father told them he knows my rights. I looked at these two sorry excuses for nurses and said, "Forget about my rights. I'm not moving. You can pull any tactic you want. I will fight you on this no matter what." At this point, I became a repeat offender of what I did back in 2012. I stood up and yelled, "Get out of my room, you poor excuse of nurses and HUMANS!" My father called my mother and said I think we need to forget about dinner tonight. That made me feel bad. Maybe I should just shut up and deal with it for his sake. My Dad wasn't having it though. To make a long story short, I never got moved. I'd like to say that the rest of this hospital stay was uneventful but again, it's me we're talking about.

So if you ever stayed in the hospital, you know that they give you socks. The kind of socks with grips on the bottom, so you don't slip. Now my feet are a size 7, the average size for a female. What the hell were they thinking when they gave me a man's XL? My sister had taken my laundry home to wash it and I was not putting my bare feet on the disgusting hospital floor. The thought of walking barefoot in the bathroom alone made me queasy. So, I put these socks on even though they hung off my feet by about three inches. The next morning at about 5:00, I had to pee badly. The sun was not up yet so my room was somewhat dark. I barely had my eyes open so I wasn't going to turn on a light. I got out of bed to walk to the bathroom. Well, you combine the darkness with me being half-asleep, plus socks way too big for my feet, guess what? Yep, I fell. Not badly. I landed against the side of the bed and on my butt. I got up right away. The only mistake I made, which I ended up regretting, is telling the doctor.

A cardiologist from my doctor's team came to see me shortly thereafter. He asked me how my morning was going. I told him I was ok except for falling. Well, he took it a lot more seriously than I did. I tried to explain that it was for the above reasons, and nothing related to dizziness from the brain surgery. He wasn't having any of it. He checked me out and then left the room. I could hear him yelling at the nurses. I truly felt bad. One of them mentioned that I was in a low-risk room. He went ape-shit. I heard him tell her that I was still a patient and needed to be watched. He came back to my room with two nurses. Now all the lights were on. He stood there while the nurses explained that I would now have a bed alarm and would have it to ring for the nurse when I had to use the bathroom. I felt like I was five years old. Now I remember what it feels like in school to raise your hand to go to the bathroom. "Is this necessary?" I asked. "Absolutely." my doctor said. "Your head has an incision. If you fall and hit your head, it can be harmful to not only where you had surgery but other parts of your body." So I spent the remainder of my hospital stay ringing for the nurse every time I needed to use the bathroom. It was humiliating.

My team of doctors suggested that a rehabilitation facility as an inpatient would be to my benefit after the hospital. It was the quickest and best way to get me back on my feet. Little did I know that it would also do a number on me mentally. The hospital recommended three facilities, one being the hospital's rehabilitation facility, one not too close, and one that was the most convenient for me and well known for its work. Of course, I went with that one. Not only did I want the best care available, but also wanted to make this as easy as possible for my family. They had to balance coming to see me with their work schedule. I didn't want to travel to make it even more stressful. Little did I know, the hospital wanted me in their facility. Not because they adored me and couldn't stand to lose me, but why else….money. If I stayed for rehab there, they could bill my insurance even more. They told me that they submitted my application to the other facility but were waiting for them to respond. Little did they know, I had connections of my own with the facility I wanted.

By connections, I mean family that worked there. I placed a phone call to that relative to see what the holdup was. I found out that the rehab facility was the one who was waiting for the hospital that is. Not only that but there was already a bed waiting with my name on it. I hung up and was mad as hell.

I rang for the nurse and when she came in, I asked her what the holdup was. Again, I was told they are waiting at the rehab place. I looked right at her and said, "Oh really? Then why did I just get off the phone with them and be advised that they are waiting for me? They also said that they are waiting for the hospital to send the paperwork. My family works there."

"Oh they do?" she asked with a dumb expression on her face. I knew it wasn't her fault. She was just following orders.

"I'll get right to it then." The nurse high-tailed out of my room. She reminded me of the Roadrunner. (laughing)

Amazingly a few minutes went by, and she came back. I was ready to go! Paperwork was sent and received. The facility was expecting me.

The discharge papers were in her hand. What a miracle! My husband drove me to the facility.

Since I did not need an IV and could walk, there was no need to travel in an ambulance for once.

Chapter 10

(2016) "And I'm the one that needs therapy?"

    Once I got to the rehab facility, I was brought right to registration which was only about ten minutes. I was told that I was getting my own room but that could change if their patient load increased. I asked if there were ever more than two people per room. The intake person looked shocked at my question. Had I not gone through what I did in the hospital, I would never think it would be something to consider. Anyway, she told me, no and I felt a sigh of relief. I was brought up to my room and immediately impressed. Except for the curtain around the bed, this also could have been a hotel room with a twin-size bed. There were some pictures on the wall, a window with a nice view and a big television. Plus, I had a whole vanity section with a sink. I had a big bathroom with a shower capable of holding two people. A duo came in a nurse and an aide. They went over items they brought to me, shampoo, soap, towels, etc. The nurse told me that my aide was there for whatever I needed. They put up "Latex Allergy" signs around the room to alert staff members. What I didn't like was that they put the bed alarm on. I explained what happened in the hospital with my fall, but the nurse told me that this was the doctor's order and they had to adhere to it. After a few days, if I prove that I can handle getting up without help, I can ask the doctor assigned to me to omit it from the order. The nurse then went over what my daily schedule and routine will be like. I was spending the next two weeks there. I'd wake up, have my vitals taken, have breakfast, then proceed to my therapy sessions. I had to travel by wheelchair only with a transporter. The sessions were one hour each daily. I was scheduled for speech, occupational and physical therapy. To this day, speech and occupational therapy proved themselves to be a waste of time for me and physical therapy is not far behind, but I'll leave that for another part of this chapter. I am sure numerous people benefit from this facility every day. It is highly reputable with strict standards. I am just not sure if it was for me.

The next morning, as previously mentioned, the staff took my blood, and my vitals, and then breakfast was served. I couldn't complain. The room was cheerful and bright, the breakfast was tasty, and their coffee was good. I was content. Plus, I still couldn't feel anything on my right side, so I didn't care if they needed a blood draw. Since I had a bed alarm, my clothes were brought over to me to change in bed. Oh! I forgot to mention that. I no longer had to wear the dreaded hospital gowns if I chose not to. I could wear my clothing. I could wear a bra too! Since I was going to be doing physical therapy, I changed into sports bras and wore tank tops and sweatpants. For the first few days, I went to Speech therapy first. The first session was an evaluation. I had to pronounce twenty words in the English language. I did ok until I got to the word "menagerie." I did not have a problem pronouncing it, I had just never heard this word before. I said "mangiare" (with an accent) because I thought maybe they were testing me and threw in an Italian word. The therapist asked me if I could recognize words in other languages. I nodded that I could, and she took the paperback with the words on it, and said, "You don't need this. There's nothing wrong with your ability to recognize words. Especially if you can recognize them in more than one language." By the way, if you don't know, according to Merriam-Webster, "menagerie" means a place where animals are kept and trained especially for the exhibition, a collection of wild or foreign animals kept especially for the exhibition or a varied mixture. I then was sent back to the waiting room for the transporter to take me back to my room or if my next session was soon thereafter, I would just be taken there. In this case, it was, and it was occupational therapy this time.

Now I am not saying that this type of therapy is not important. Many people need it and require it. My daughter attends grad school to major in it. It just wasn't for me. At least not the therapy I received. Maybe this is why the medical field gets a bad rap. I had a stroke in 2014. I very much could have used all these therapies to get back on track; especially working with hands for occupational therapy. But you are sent to therapy based on what you're being discharged from the hospital with. The stroke left me with my speech slurred and not able to swallow. I walked with a limp and my right hand was numb. Therapy was never mentioned. This time around in 2016, I had brain surgery, so I was sent to the brain injury wing of the facility.

I had already been talking clearly for over a year and could swallow and exercised a little each day. But the hospital listed all these different therapies as part of my recovery from the brain surgery. I didn't know any better. So anyway, I get to occupational therapy. The therapist hands me a paper filled with different photos of what's normally in a standard bathroom. She tells me to study the paper for about thirty seconds, then turns it over. I then must proceed to tell her as many things I can in thirty seconds that were on the paper. The purpose of it is to study if I suffered any functional cognitive impairments. Meaning if I needed support in functioning on how to bathe, brush my teeth, etc. I felt humiliated and embarrassed that this may be how people are perceiving me to be. I glared at the young therapist "Seriously? Is this a joke?" Because I won't remember or think to say toilet, sink, tub? C'mon!" I went on to tell her that not only do I know how to brush my teeth, but I follow up with flossing and mouthwash. Needless to say, I passed and was now on my way to physical therapy.

Physical therapy may have been beneficial because it was exercise and got my joints moving rather than being in bed all day. However, I still managed to get scolded. I was put on a stationary bike and told to peddle. The bike tracked my heart rate and speed. I guess I was overdoing it because another therapist who wasn't assigned to me, saw me and tattled on me. Didn't they ever hear of "snitches get stitches?" My therapist told me to slow down. On the second day, I woke up and ate my breakfast. I had a session in fifteen minutes, yet my transporter hadn't arrived. They are supposed to arrive at least twenty minutes before a session. He finally showed up, got me in the wheelchair, and off we went. We waited in the elevator for over ten minutes. The whole facility uses wheelchairs and only three fit into 1 of the three elevators at a time so there was usually a wait. The analog clock was behind me so I couldn't see the time. If you miss your session you have to reschedule for a later time in the day. I did not want to do that. I was up, dressed, had visitors coming later, and just wanted to get this over with. I asked the orderly what the time was. His response was, I kid you not. "Oh, I can't read that type of clock Ma'am. Only digital."

I turned my head back around, bit my lip, and thought to myself, "And I'm the one that needs therapy?" (laughing)

I am now in my second session of speech

therapy. The young therapist explains the routine to me. Guess what? It is exactly what they did in the hospital. I swallow water and applesauce while she feels my throat to see how well it went down. I told her all of this was done two years ago and nothing came of it. "I eat normally, just taking it easy when I drink since my throat can only handle a little bit of liquid at a time." She just nodded so I continued. "My vocal cord is paralyzed from the stroke. I receive botulinum injections for Achalasia disorder. Swallowing may come back one day, and it may not. All the voice exercises and such won't change that. I know how to properly pronounce words in English, Italian and Spanish. I am sorry. I just feel this is a waste of your time, my time, and my insurance company's money." She told me to humor her and do the test anyway. So, I complied but not before rolling my eyes. Guess what happened next? I was discharged from Speech.

Next, I went to Occupational Therapy. It was more time wasted. This day was a group session, meaning other patients will be in my session. The therapist asks us if we know where we are. Again, I roll my eyes. Of course, I know where I am! I am not senile. I would prefer to be at home, however. She asks me first and I tell her the correct location. I bend my head down in disbelief because I can't believe I am away from my family for this, and my insurance company is paying the bill for this nonsense. The therapist continues and asks the patient next to me. He responds with a town about thirty minutes away. Now granted he was elderly but c'mon! I did not belong here with these patients. Speech and Occupational can kiss it when it comes to me!

At least my next session was physical therapy and there were exercises I could not do. That's where I needed to spend my time. I ended up having one more occupational therapy session where we played Uno and had to plan a vacation.

"That's it," I said. "This is a joke. I play Uno regularly with my kids-(I just played it the other night and beat my son!)-Also, I just planned a whole vacation for this coming November since the doctor said I will be healed by then. I lost my hearing on my right side and have some balance issues that I need to work on. How is this possibly helping? My mind was never an issue. It might be, however, if I continue this." The therapist looked stunned. I felt bad. You could tell she just graduated recently and was new to working with patients. But now my time and money were being taken advantage of and I wasn't having it. I was discharged from OT.

After being discharged from Speech and OT, I had extra time on my hands during the day. While any other day, I would welcome this, here the days were long and boring. I only had visitors, meals, and showers to look forward to. A man came to see me. He said he was the event organizer for the patients and wanted to introduce himself. They had activities and events each week to make the patients happy and keep them occupied. He took me in my wheelchair down the hall to the computer room. Little did I know it would become my best friend for the next ten days. It had the internet and Wi-Fi! He told me about an event they were having the following day, a casino. If interested, I was to let my nurse know so she could arrange for a transporter to pick me up and take me. That night I grabbed single dollars from whatever family came to see me. I was excited and would attend this event right after therapy, then I'd follow up with some social media. By the time that was all over, it would be time for dinner and visitors.

The next day, after therapy, I gobbled down my lunch, washed my face, and rang for the transporter to take me to the casino event. I've been to Vegas and Atlantic City. I knew it obviously would be nothing like that, but I've been to enough Italian Feasts also to know how a casino event is run and orchestrated. The orderly brought me to a cafeteria-type of room. The event was not what I expected. I did not know whether to laugh or cry. The organizer was sitting at a long table with a few elderly patients. He motioned for the transporter to bring me over. On the table were toy horses. The kind you buy for your kids to put in their toy barns, about 4-5 inches each. They all had a string attached to them. Each patient had to pull their horse along the table. The first one to reach the end wins. I was shocked but amused. Hey, I had some money, so why not? These senior citizens got nothing on me!

I pulled out my singles and Bob, the organizer says, "Oh no, you don't need that. We play with fake money." My jaw dropped. Is this dude for real? But he was sincere, so I played along. After ten minutes or so, I was over it. I lied and said my head was beginning to throb and I was tired. They rang for the transporter, and I wheeled myself out into the hallway. I waited and waited, with no orderly. So, I wheeled to the elevator and put myself in. I got to my floor, got out and my nurse saw me. She asked where the transporter was, and I threw my hands in the air. She told me I cannot travel by myself and to just wait in that spot while she got someone to take me back to my room. Again, I waited and waited, but no one came. "This is ridiculous." "How about I give myself some physical therapy of my own and wheel myself down the hallway?" It took me a few tries to learn how to maneuver the wheelchair, but I got the hang of it and wheeled away. I wheeled myself to the nurse's station which is the midpoint between the elevator and my room. The nurses looked at me and I smiled. Just as one of them was opening her mouth to speak, probably to ask me how I got there, I asked if one of them could put me in the computer room which is just on the other side of their station. A nurse wheeled me over to a computer where I spent the next three hours.

When I could no longer feel my fingers, I decided to go back to my room. An elderly woman was in her wheelchair right outside just sitting in the hallway. She said hello to me and asked me if I could hang out with her for a while. She was lonely. It broke my heart. So, I did. She introduced herself, telling me her name was Mary, and told me she had two daughters around my age. One of them had not spoken to her in five years and the other one told her she will try to visit but probably won't. She went on to tell me about the relationships she had with each of her daughters. It was pretty non-existent. Her husband passed away a few years back from a heart attack. She just had brain surgery and had no one to rely on, to visit her, or anything else. My heart went out to her. I sat there, in the hallway for as long as I could. My stomach began to rumble, and I knew my parents would be there soon. I politely excused myself but promised to visit her in her room around the same time tomorrow. I wheeled back to my room but had tears in my eyes. This is probably the most vulnerable position a person can be in, and it sucks to have to do it alone. I thought of my own life. Eventually, my parents won't be here, and what if my husband isn't either like Mary's? What if my kids have an estranged relationship with me? I didn't want to think about my future, so I turned on the television. Luckily my dinner came soon thereafter, followed by my parents.

By now, the bed alarm was getting on my

nerves. They didn't want me out of bed by myself, yet I could wheel myself all over because the transporter doesn't show up and no one blinks an eye? That morning I had to pee badly. I rang for the aid. Five minutes later, I rang again. No one still. By this point, I was squirming. If you had a stroke, you may know this. There is little control one may have within their body. Because I could not feel in certain places, it was difficult to hold my bladder. I jumped out of bed, sending the bed alarm wailing. I rushed into the bathroom and felt a sigh of relief. A few moments later, I hear an aide asking me if I'm ok. I wash my hands and then open the door.

The aide is standing there with a concerned look on her face. She proceeds to tell me that I am supposed to ring for someone and that I have a bed alarm. No shit! I tell her calmly that I did, TWICE and that no one came. She tells me I have to wait then. "Don't go getting anyone in trouble." "Really? Is that what she cared about? I wanted to punch her. It took every bit of me to not ask her if she felt like changing my urine-drenched sheets after if that was the case and that I don't give a shit if you get reprimanded or not, guess what, it's your job Bitch." However, I smiled and said I won't report anyone. That's not my style but someone needs to answer the call when I ring." I had enough of the nasty people that I've had to deal with. I will probably never see these people again, God willing. It wasn't worth my stress.

Something I guess I had to learn for myself as I got older and wiser. That same night, it happened again. No one came so I went myself. As history repeats itself often, I got the same spiel only it was a different aid this time. The result: they took the bed alarm off.

In the end, I spent two weeks there before being discharged. I told Mary that I would keep in touch, calling and writing to her when I could. I called the phone number she had given me. A woman answered, probably one of her estranged daughters. Mary had passed away a few weeks prior. I still wasn't allowed to drive and she was buried in a cemetery that was two hours away. I couldn't visit the gravesite and pay my respects. I hope you're in a happier place now, Mary.

Chapter 11

(2016) "Where do they find these people?"

Have you ever seen the Richard Bey Show? I'm probably aging myself when I ask that. It was a popular talk show in the 90s. Richard Bey was the host and famous for asking, "Where do they find these people?" He would ask that when he had a guest that told an unimaginable or outrageous story of what their life was like, how they acted, etc. Once I got home and continued my therapy as an outpatient, I found myself asking the very same thing.

Part of my recovery and healing involved home therapy. Even though I was discharged from occupational therapy at the rehab facility, the doctor ordered services for me to have at home. Its purpose was to help me settle back into physical, daily life activities such as bathing, going up and down my stairs, etc. First I had physical therapy. It wasn't too bad, it got me daily exercise. Still, it was nothing that I couldn't do on my own. The therapist took my temperature, blood pressure, and heart rate. I can do those things. I even own a blood pressure machine. And as far as the exercises go, I sat in a chair and raised my legs. Isn't it more effort to walk down the stairs to open the door when she comes and to climb them once I let her in? And did they know how much online shopping I do? I am best friends with Amazon. Something is always left on my doorstep that I must go fetch. I ended up having three sessions before being discharged.

Then there was occupational therapy. Once again, this was a joke. The dude that came to my house was an older man. He carried a bag of tools with him. He climbed my steps but stopped on each of my seventeen stairs, to rest his bag. My mother and I just looked at each other. I whispered, "I think he is the one that needs therapy." He sat down, breathing heavily, and started pulling things out of his bag. He wanted me to squeeze a sponge, telling me I needed to do this daily for my hand. Look, I'm no doctor, but I didn't sprain or break my hand. It is paralyzed from the stroke. All the squeezing and moving of my hand isn't going to bring back my nerves if they don't want to come back. It has been over six years since the stroke as I write this. I've washed many, many dishes and cleaned my house, squeezing sponges. The feeling in my right hand, yeah I got nothing. But, he was here and my insurance company was being billed for this visit no matter what, so I played along, squeezing the sponge.

Next, he whipped out a catalog. It contained all sorts of tools to help disabled people function in the home. He flipped to the bathroom section and showed me a back brush, similar to what you would find in your local drug store. He suggested I purchase one. Like I said earlier. Maybe all of this should have been addressed when I had the stroke, not after the brain surgery that affected my hearing and balance.

Even though I didn't want or need one I asked him why I would pay about twenty dollars more for this one in the catalog rather than one from the drug store. He told me that the one in the catalog is longer, making it easier to reach. I politely said, "Ok, but I'm good." Then he wanted me to look at chairs for the shower. Is this guy for real? Was he an occupational therapist or a salesman for the catalog company? I could not wait for the session to be over. It was a complete waste of time. Upon leaving, he wanted to schedule my next appointment. I said, "Uh, I don't know what my week looks like yet. I'll call the office to schedule." I never made another appointment. But I continue to take showers, STANDING and washing my back.

The following week I got a phone call from a hearing aid company. They explained that they received my information from the hospital, knew about my surgery, and wanted to discuss the products they offer to improve my hearing in my right ear. Again, does anyone know anything about the fields they work in? I told the representative on the phone that if she could bring back my hearing in my right ear, I will buy the most expensive model and give her a hefty commission because there was no way my hearing was coming back unless you gave me a whole new head. She hung up on me. (laughing)

When I was in the rehab facility, the director talked with me about applying for Social Security benefits. She told me that I am a candidate for it and I should try. I had to think about that. It was getting harder and harder to work. I was getting older for starters. The stroke did a number on me. It was hard driving home in the dark, my hand would go numb when I typed on my work computer, and had trouble walking. The business I was in had me on a phone call for an hour or so at times. It would be difficult to do that with hearing in one ear only since I would not be able to switch the receiver from ear to ear. I could just imagine the pain from my neck to my shoulder down my arm on my left side that would develop from using one side only. Plus, if two people were talking to me at once, I often became confused and flustered. My head would throb. I already mentioned the vocal cord issue. Sometimes when I speak, a word or two come out of me as though I'm yelling at the person even though I'm not. I didn't want to come off as rude if it wasn't intentional.

My husband and I had several long discussions about whether I should stop working and collect disability or keep working. There was so much to consider. Being financially stable was important obviously. We had to compare what I was making from a paycheck versus what Social Security Department (SSD) would pay. I could eliminate weekly gas fill-ups and having to order lunch from my expenses if I stopped working. I also would not pay the work premium for medical insurance.

But what about health insurance? SSD enrolls you in Medicare after two years of having benefits, but I had a heart condition. Could I wait two years? Forget, paying Cobra. That was way too expensive. I could buy a plan but the more they covered, the higher the premium. I had an echocardiogram every year. That alone has a high price! Also, you're paid monthly if you're on SSD. Could I discipline and budget myself so that I covered myself for an entire month? It meant I would always be around for the kids, however, and that was huge. They did so much in school.

They often had to turn things down because we couldn't get them to an activity or pick them up. But I couldn't forget that this was even a sure thing. I still had to apply. I have heard stories of people being denied for one reason or another with Social Security.

But what the hell? I was on sick leave from work for three months. I was receiving short-term disability payments already so I had some time to work on this before I had to return to work and some money to tie me over if I wasn't going to return. I started the process immediately.

Going to the Social Security office was an experience. One that I would rather forget. I could have applied online but so many official documents and records were required. I was not comfortable mailing my whole history anywhere. Plus I wanted to meet in person. I wanted that office to see me and know that I had legitimate issues and not just some loser that wanted to not work and live off the system.

The office itself was situated in the middle of a bad neighborhood. My father insisted on going with me as the neighborhood had a high crime rate. The office was no better. The customers there looked so helpless and pitiful that I was concerned that I may look too good to be able to receive benefits. I probably waited about an hour to be seen, even though I had an appointment. I felt like a degenerate waiting there. The people there either looked like some sort of mutant or were there simply to milk the system even though they had no business being on Social Security. But then again, the same might be said about me.

After what felt like an eternity, my name was

called, and my father and I walked over to a desk. The first question asked was if I speak English and could understand it. "Yes, that is not a problem," unlike the woman at the desk next to mine who did not understand a word they said!

I was asked if I feel like I am entitled to benefits and why? What health issues did I have? Had this dude not been sitting, I would have told him to pull up a chair. I had a long medical history. If the rest of these people could get disability, so could I.

He then told me if I'm awarded benefits, I could not work for wages while on it. Do you understand what that means?" *Did he just ask me that?* In my head, I was like, *Seriously dude?* Isn't that why I am here in the first place and you're asking me if I understand? C'mon!

But, unfortunately, many people are dishonest and always look for a meal ticket. Plus, I did not want to piss this man off since nothing could stop him from tossing my application in the garbage so I simply mumbled, "yes."

After the interview process, my father dropped me off at home. I knew that I did everything I could to have benefits rewarded. I submitted my entire medical history, financials, and everything else besides my firstborn. It was up to God and the government now. The SSD representative told me it could take 3-4 months to come to a decision. My file had to be reviewed.

Like I said earlier, I had 3 months off from work before I had to return or I could lose my job. I prayed a decision would be reached by then. But what if I was declined? Then what? I did have legitimate issues. Could I handle the stress of going back to work each day mentally and physically? My brain hurts now when I get confused. My hand throbs when I use a writing instrument for more than a few minutes. Sometimes, I can't even put my earrings in, my hand becomes so numb. I prayed.

Three months came and went. I checked every day both online and in my mailbox. Every time I logged in online, it just read. "In progress."

I was nearing the date to return to work. I called my supervisor. I worked with her for fifteen years and we had a good relationship with each other. She was tight with the head of the company and often sat in on meetings with the Human Resources department. I asked her if she would consider extending my medical leave a little longer. I was honest with her and told her after that, there is a chance I might not return. There were too many issues now. When she told me that it was fine by her, my position was being covered, I asked her to gently break the news to the rest of management and I will officially request an extension. This wasn't a problem. I felt a sigh of relief and prayed again that the decision would come.

About two weeks later, I was hanging out in the driveway with my husband and kids. The weather was starting to change and it was nice out. We were planting flowers on our lawn. The mailman pulled up and my husband walked over to him to grab the mail. He looked through the pile of mail, mostly junk and whatnot. Then as I was bent over, arranging some Impatiens in the dirt, I heard my husband say in a smirky tone, "Oh Stacy. There's a letter from Social Security here." I jumped up and grabbed the envelope from him. I did the Sign of the Cross and ripped open the envelope. Inside was a letter addressed to me. The first line read, "Congratulations, you have been awarded Social Security benefits." I began to cry. For the first time in my life, I felt like there was some type of recompense for all I had been through. Someone took notice. Not that I ever felt entitled to anything because I did not. I just needed a break from it all and something good to come out of all this. I hugged my family and told them what the letter stated and that I was going to call my job in the morning to resign. Now all I had to do was figure out how to get through the next two years without health insurance. But there would be no more sitting in traffic daily, dealing with snotty coworkers and rude people on the phone. More importantly, I would be there when my kids came home from school each day and my husband would come home to a clean house and a warm home-cooked meal each night.

I spent the next month or two always looking over my shoulder. There was always a concern that someone from Social Security was spying on me to make sure I am disabled. What if I walked too fast or was carrying something heavy? These are just some of the things that went through my mind, daily. I heard stories of the person who hurt their back at work or some other body part and was collecting benefits and compensation.

"Relax," someone told me. "They don't look at people like you. You have legitimate problems that are internal. Sorry, but those problems aren't going away. It's Joe Shmo, who claims he hurt his finger at work and needs to be out for a year that they watch. Not you." I felt better but was still leery about it.

It didn't help that at the time I was reading an article about Social Security Fraud. Many law enforcement officials claimed they suffered from something in the 9/11 attacks. They were collecting benefits while earning wages somewhere else or engaging in activities one could not do if their physical injury was legit. One was even caught selling cannoli at the San Gennaro Feast! Hanno un ottimo sapore!

The head of Human Resources from my place of employment contacted me. She said they couldn't force me but as an act of good faith, it is their policy for an employee to have an exit interview. Even though my case was pretty clear and I was leaving for medical reasons, there was a form to fill out about why I was resigning. I agreed to it. After all, they did extend my medical leave and were cooperative throughout this whole ordeal. I made an appointment for the following week.

Upon arrival at the office, I went straight to the management's suite. I had my interview with staff members from H.R. as well as my supervisor. I explained why I was leaving and thanked them for all they'd done. The management themselves never did much for me other than cut me a paycheck each week. However, I busted my ass daily for them, so I earned it and didn't feel an ounce of sympathy or regret.

As for my supervisor, she did more, working with me when I had to leave work early to care for my niece, extend medical leaves, etc. But, I thanked them all because I don't believe in burning bridges. I walked out of there with a smile on my face.

Before I left the building, I decided to stop by my department. There were a few coworkers that I liked and wanted to say goodbye to. Some of them spent more hours with me daily for the last fifteen years than I did with my husband. I may or may not have had a working wife.

Anyway, I was greeted with open arms. Some of my coworkers seemed genuine when asking how I'd been and that they missed me. All of them asked me when I was returning. I told them I wasn't. I just had a close-out interview with management and I was here to say goodbye and take any personal belongings I had left there before going out on leave. Most of them were supportive, wishing me well and telling me they understood. One coworker however came across a little differently. Maybe she didn't mean it the way she said it, yet I still wanted to slap her. She proceeds to say with a grimaced look on her face, "I wish I could stay home and have the government pay me." I turned and looked dead into her eyes. "Well," I said, biting my lip to hold back the urge to tell her to kiss my ass, "I paid a heavy price for this. If I had my choice, I'd rather be healthy and keep on working. I think we can all agree that being lazy is just not who I am. I always gave 100% to my work duties, sometimes even picking up the slack for those who didn't work to their full capacity. " I then winked at the bitch. One of my other coworkers, kind of like a second mom to me, wraps her arms around me, kisses me on the cheek, and tells me she loves me. With that, I grab my stuff, say "Ciao" to everyone, blow kisses, and out the door, I went. I was ready to end this chapter of my life and start a new one.

Chapter 12

(2016-2017) "Follow the Leader"

Over the next two years, I adjusted to being a full-time wife, mom, and housekeeper. my kids were not babies, so I was not the exhausted new mom or crazed with little ones running around. Still, as much as I loved being home, I needed a purpose in my life, something other than just the matriarch of the family. Even though my husband and the life we built is my greatest accomplishment, I yearned for something that was me and me alone. When I worked, I took pride in my work. If something physically or hypothetically had my name on it, I gave it my all. Gianna would be going to college soon. Frankie was starting high school and certainly didn't need his Mommy up his ass all the time and Mia was about to start kindergarten. Without kids in the house at all for most of the day, what would I do with myself? I was not the Peg Bundy type, sitting on the couch all day, watching tv, eating snacks. That summer I thought about this daily. All the kids were home for the summer so I was preoccupied but what will happen when they go back? Mia's school was holding an orientation for incoming kindergartners, in late August of that year. I registered with her on the day of the orientation. Even though I was familiar with the school from my older kids, Mia was not and I wanted her to know it somewhat before starting the school year so she didn't freak out.

Walking down the hallway towards the auditorium where the orientation was beginning, I passed a Girl Scout table. The recruiter at the table stopped me. "Would you be interested in signing your daughter up to be a Girl Scout?: She asked. I bent down to look at Mia and asked her. She nodded and smiled. The recruiter lady told me they are trying to form a new troop. There were other girls interested in joining but they were looking for an adult leader to run it. "Would you be interested in becoming a leader? she asked me. My first reaction was to say no. I had too many issues to be running after a bunch of 5-6-year-olds. I wrote down my info and told the lady to contact me if she does find a leader and a troop is formed. I would be interested in registering Mia. I walked away toward the auditorium, holding Mia's hand.

During the presentation, I could not stop thinking about being a leader. Could I do it? I did not work anymore, and I used to dream of being a teacher. This would be similar to the number of hours, number of kids, and having a boss with coworkers. But no paycheck! However, I did tell the man above that if he spared me my life after having a stroke and a brain tumor and I could live a normal one, then I would spend the rest of it doing good deeds and helping others. I thought dedicating my time to influence, encourage and educate little ladies in life and to be good people was a great way to do just that. Plus, it meant getting involved in an extracurricular activity with my youngest. Something I never got to do with my other two. When orientation was over, I stopped back at the Girl Scout table and told the recruiter to sign me up as a leader and enroll my daughter in my troop. She would be my first scout! I don't know who was more excited, the recruiter, Mia, or myself!

As the days followed, I did all the necessary training and filled out paperwork and such. Now I just had to wait. I was told I need at least four girls to form a troop. But, that shouldn't be too difficult, the Girl Scout recruiter had told me. Many kindergartners were waiting for troops. That wasn't the problem.

Finding an adult to be a leader is. Soon thereafter, one by one, a girl signed up. Within two weeks after I registered as a leader, I had a full troop. I am not going to lie. As much as I wanted to do this, I did not want to deal with psychotic families. This was something I was doing to bring both myself, my daughter, and maybe other little girls, joy, and happiness. Every time I got an email with the little girl's name, I stalked the parent's Facebook for any info I could

231

get to form an opinion of them. I didn't need any other drama in my life. If they looked off, I was walking! However, I would come across photos of what I assumed were the new scouts. They were adorable and I felt an instant connection with them. I knew I had to do this, I was meant to do it and I promised I'd give it my all. Once we became official, I did just that.

The Community recruiter suggested I start holding meetings one to two months after school started. Since the girls were just starting kindergarten, she advised allowing time to let them transition to that before beginning scouting. I agreed to this. I had to transition myself! I needed to look at the different meetings I could do, forms that families had to sign, set up a social media page to post information, and more! I set a goal to make this be one awesome troop, one that each girl, including myself, could be proud of.

The day finally arrived to have my first meeting. I was so excited. I was even excited to dress Mia from head to toe in the Girl Scout uniform. I found Girl Scout snack bars in the grocery store one morning. I was bringing those along with my personal Keurig. My meeting was at the local library. I was setting up a table for the parents to help themselves to coffee and snacks. I wanted the first meeting to feel welcoming to all. For the girls, I had balloons, snacks, candy, and more. I even downloaded Girl Scout songs to my phone to play softly in the background.

That morning started as normal. I saw my two older kids off to school and then got Mia ready for school herself. As soon as she got on the bus, I was planning on going over everything I had for the meeting to make sure nothing was forgotten. My day did not go according to plan.

After I put Mia on the bus, I walked into the kitchen. My cat, Stella, was pushing a Yankee Candle across the kitchen counter. "Knock it off, before you knock it off, Stell," I told my kitty as if she understood me. As soon as I turned my back, I heard the crash. Glass scattered all over as the candle broke from the fall. Stella took off like a bat out of hell. Hence the term, Scaredy Cat. I swept up the broken glass, then vacuumed to make sure I got it all. Afterward, I sat down to print some final paperwork for the meeting. My printer jammed and several blank pieces of paper with splattered ink marks on them came out when I fixed the printer. Since they were now useless, I walked over to the garbage to toss them.

My garbage pail was filled almost to the top but not quite. I pushed the paper down to make more room to fit more garbage before we brought the bag outside.

Getting back to the stroke, remember when I said I had numbness and then right-sided weakness? My nerves have a delayed reaction when there is any type of sensation on my right side. I've been burned a few times by reaching into the oven when it's on. Anyway, I pushed my right hand down to squash the paper down, forgetting that I threw the bigger pieces of glass right in the garbage while I swept the little shards into a paper bag. As soon as I started to take my hand off the top of the paper, I felt it. I knew something bad just happened. I looked at my hand and blood began to spurt. I quickly turned on my sink to wash the wound. The blood just kept seeping out. I grabbed paper towels to soak up the blood and put pressure on the wound. I called my husband because I didn't know what to do. I described what happened and he told me I need to call an ambulance. I probably need stitches. I called my parents and they told me the same thing. My father insisted on coming to my house. I called 911 next and explained my emergency. I was told to keep pressure on the wound until EMS got there. I said ok and hung up. I passed a mirror in my house. I forgot it was still the morning. I did not shower, my hair was a mess and I had no bra on! I ran into my bedroom to at least put on a bra. I left drops of blood throughout my house. The only good thing about this was since I had a minimal feeling, I wasn't in pain. I could hear the sirens coming up the road. I opened my front door to find the local sheriff walking past my house to see which house he needed to go to. I'm glad I wasn't being raped or anything! I waved him down. He must have been a rookie sheriff because he did not look much older than my Gianna.

"What's the problem Ma'am?" he asked me as if I steered him away from something important. 911 doesn't brief the police on the scene they're about to encounter? I wondered. Ridiculous. What if there was a man with a gun? Shouldn't the officer have a heads-up? Or was this dude just being an ass? I started to tell him what just transpired when the fire department's ambulance and the hospital ambulance pulled up. At least they had the right house! "Now we have a party," I said as I found this whole scene to be exaggerated and so extra.

An older gentleman from the fire ambulance looked at my hand and said, "Let's get you cleaned up." Now we're were getting somewhere. I walked back into my house with him followed by a younger gentleman that also came from the fire ambulance, two EMS workers, and the sheriff. I was told to sit on my couch and my hand was wrapped up. The sheriff told me he had to take a report and tell him what happened. I know it's protocol and this young ass was just following the procedure, but I still thought of it as a waste of time. I told him anyway. The older gentleman told me he wrapped up the wound but I would need a stitch or two. I had to go to the hospital.

"Can I wait for my husband?" I asked him as I thought about my meeting. The man looked right at me." I wouldn't. That's a pretty nasty cut and with your heart issues, you can't risk bacteria getting into the wound." Been there, done that, so I grabbed my coat. He continued speaking. "You can either ride with us or the official ambulance. But we're free." He smiled. We don't even take your insurance info. The thought of being in an ambulance made me cringe and riding alone made it even worse, but it had to be done. "I'll go with you." I smiled back.

The hospital is about a fifteen-minute ride

from my house. The ambulance takes five. At that time I learned the driver knew my daughter and was a year older. "So, you have had your driver's license for about two years and now you're driving an ambulance? Kill me now Lord." I thought as I prayed that I would arrive at the hospital in one piece. I did arrive safely, and these two kind men brought me in and stayed with me until the hospital staff took me away to examine me.

After I explained what had happened again for the fourth time that day, the doctor on call told me he could either put the stitches in or I could wait for the specialist. I did not want a botched job on my hand and I just knew this would affect my heart somehow so I opted for the latter. I waited and waited. My husband arrived at the hospital and waited with me. The doctor came back in to check on me. "How much longer? I have a meeting that I need to be at."

"I don't know when the plastic surgeon will get here. He's in surgery. It's not a big deal to put in a stitch. Even our nurses can do it. I've done it many times. I could do it now if you want to get out of here." I looked at my husband. "What do you think?" He put his hand on my shoulder. "I'm sure you will be fine but it's up to you." I sighed. "What the hell. Let's do it." Five stitches and twenty minutes later, I was out of there.

As soon as my hubby pulled into the driveway, I ran into the house. I found my poor dad in his work suit, on the floor, trying to clean up my bloody droplets. "Leave it, Dad. I'll do it when I get back. I have to jump in the shower." He looked at me like I had two heads.

"You aren't still thinking about holding the meeting, are you? You just went through some trauma. You need to rest."

"I'll rest when I'm dead," I said as I started peeling off my socks.

"Right now, can you blow up some balloons and look for Mia's bus?" He shook his head at me but agreed. Thanks, Dad! Nothing was stopping me from having this meeting. I took the quickest shower ever, threw on some jeans, and put on my shoes. I needed to pack the car. "How are you going to carry everything with stitches in one hand?" my father asked with concern. My husband had to stay behind to get my son off the bus. "I'll figure it out," I told him as I picked up the Keurig. "You won't be able to drive either." He responded with. "Well, you could take me if you're not busy," I said with a smirk. We filled his trunk with all my meeting materials.

We pulled up to the library. "Just pull up in front and let me out so you don't have to park and I won't have to walk." I jiggled my seatbelt to take it off. "No, no, no. You can't carry all this." He pulled into a space, got out, and started unloading the car. If things had not gone wrong already, it was about to become worse. My meeting was on the second floor of the library. Guess what? The elevator was out of order.

In addition to every other ailment that I had as a result of the stroke, I couldn't walk up or down a flight of stairs without holding on to the railing. Combine that with not being able to carry anything in my hand since I had stitches, yeah I was pretty useless. My father told me to head up to the room and take it slow. I told him there was way too much for him to carry by himself and especially having to do it taking the stairs. "Don't worry about me. Just be careful walking up to them. Make sure you hold on." I headed upstairs and began to set up. My father ended up making three trips up and down the stairs, carrying stuff. I could see the beads of sweat on his forehead. He had to be dying wearing a suit as well. I don't think I will ever forget that image of him. I felt terrible but also incredibly blessed to have the Father I did.

So, my journey as a Girl Scout troop leader began that day. My co-leader arrived and started complaining about her rough day and joked that we should appreciate the fact that she was there. I laughed. "You think you had a rough day? I just came from the Emergency Room. And my Father here just did three trips up and down those steps carrying all that you see here." Her jaw dropped. "What, the Emergency Room, why?"

"I'll explain later. Let's begin the meeting." I turned to look at the adorable little ladies in front of me. "Hello. I'm Miss Stacy."

Being a troop leader took much of my time because I allowed it to and was dedicated to being a good one. The girls, their families, and especially my Mia, depended on me to lead them in a positive, educated yet fun way. It was therapy for my soul too. It kept me busy, now that I no longer worked full time or any time for that matter. My kids were in school all day also. Plus, it kept my mind off thinking about why I was home all the time now. I knew in my heart that I was doing a good thing even if no one else did.

My stitches were due to come out in about 2 weeks. My husband and I planned a trip to Punta Cana then. I would go in between my biweekly troop meetings so as not to miss any. I needed a break after the way, this year went down. At one point, I thought I'd have a mental breakdown. I emailed my doctor a few days before I was going away to ask him to prescribe a diuretic for me since I tend to suffer from edema when I eat out. My Dominican friends have told me that the food cooked there has a lot of sazón and sofrito. In other words, it is high in sodium.

My doctor called me right then asking when my trip was. "It's in a few days." There was a brief silence and then he spoke. "Stacy, I do not recommend you travel right now. You have a wound that is still healing and is prone to infection. If it gets infected, you will have to be treated there. You don't want that. Especially with your medical history. It's too risky." Now I was the silent one. I then told my doctor that my plans were already made and that I will keep my hand covered from any exposure. Plus the saltwater from the ocean might do it some good. "At least let me prescribe an antibiotic to protect you from infection," he said. "Agreed." I have to admit. It did give me some relief knowing that I would be protected. In the end, we had a fabulous trip, and my hand was fine.

2017 was as normal as it could be for someone with my issues. My eldest daughter was now a senior in high school. If you have ever had a senior in high school before, you know it's a busy time. There are all the senior nights if they have been involved in school extracurricular activities, college applications, and their open houses, preparing for graduation, and then there's the prom. Multiply the time you will spend on all things prom if you have a daughter. We're talking, about the dress, makeup, hair, and then, of course, the date! Has anyone ever heard of a promposal before? Was that even a thing back in my day? My daughter and I had numerous conversations over ideas for her to ask this boy she wanted to take to the prom. Both my daughter and this boy were avid hockey players, so she wanted her proposal to reflect hockey there somewhere. She finally settled on making a sign, spelling out "Prom?" on roller hockey wheels on the ground. She presented this to him after one of his games at the rink. He said "Yes."

From there, we scoped out makeup artists and went dress shopping. We have a family member that does our hair, so that was already decided upon beforehand. At least it was one thing we didn't have to do. The day of the prom arrived and Gianna looked like a supermodel. From head to toe, she was glamorous. Her date stood there in awe when he first laid eyes on her.

A month later she graduated with honors. She still hadn't decided on what she wanted to major in so she would work and attend the community college until she figured out what she wanted to do. As for my other two children, they went through the motions of a regular school year, both doing well.

That summer, we took our usual family trip. My parents, my sister, my nieces, and us. My younger niece was pregnant, and we were so excited. Mia was six by then and it was time to have a new baby in the family. Two-piece bathing suits were not a part of my world anymore. I had gained a lot of weight. Something I thought I'd never have to deal with. It was the one perk I had from having a heart condition. It kept me thin. My parents were concerned about my ever-growing body. They shot looks and made comments when I reached for the bread on the table or ordered a second drink. I know it was out of concern, but it just added to how I already was feeling with all my issues.

As fall was approaching that year, I was eager to start the routine of getting the kids ready for school and begin to plan my Girl Scout meetings. This gave me purpose in life. I wouldn't just be some disabled the woman that sits on the couch all day and lets the system take care of her. The holidays were good that year, normal. But as 2018 was around the corner, I started to sweat.

Chapter 13

(2018-2019) "Did I just run a marathon?"

As I mentioned earlier, something awful happened to me medically every two years and it was in the even years, beginning with 2006. I had a miscarriage in 2006, open heart surgery in 2008, followed by another miscarriage in 2010. 2012 was another open heart surgery from the infection. Then there was the mother of them all, a stroke in 2014. In 2016, the brain tumor was removed and I caught pneumonia from it. So now that 2018 was here, I was on edge. I kept all my doctor appointments and tried watching what I ate but did not attempt to start a new diet. I was doing everything I could to prevent anything from happening to my body.

That year came and went. "The curse is over!" I screamed in my head once the ball dropped on New Year's Eve. The year had been pretty normal. Gianna transferred to another college to further her education, Frankie made his Confirmation while Mia made her Communion. I went to the gym daily to increase my strength and endurance. My Girl Scout troop bridged from daisies to brownies that year also. So, with all these milestones happening, I stayed busy. Plus, we took the kids to Walt Disney World that summer. Life was good.

Even 2019 looked like nothing was going to happen to me health-wise. As silly as this may sound, I wasn't too concerned because it had been three years now, not two, so I convinced myself that I was good to go. We were planning a trip to Mexico with the kids so I was excited about that, I had dropped a few pounds from my daily workouts in the gym so I was delighted to wear a bikini. This would be the first time my children would see another country so I was excited for them as well. We had an amazing time and once we got back, I got us ready to begin a new school year.

Once we returned home, I started noticing my ankles were always swelling. I assumed it was from the food I had in Mexico. It was probably loaded with sodium. I called the doctor to ask for a diuretic. It helped somewhat but I noticed my stomach was expanding also. At first, I immediately thought of pregnancy. "There's no way." Plus we shared a room with the kids while in Mexico so I knew nothing took place then. If I was pregnant, I had to be at least two months anyhow for my stomach to expand like that. I ran to the drug store to buy a pregnancy test. Like I thought, it was negative. Years ago, I would have been disappointed but not this time. My life was hectic enough and I was old! But if I wasn't pregnant, what else was happening?

As the days went on, I found it harder and harder to breathe. There was pressure in my abdomen making it difficult to sit or lie down and be comfortable. My stomach was huge and hard to the touch. I was miserable. There were also times when I felt my heart racing. It was sporadic though and didn't last very long. My Fitbit was constantly showing a high heart rate and I could feel it. I felt as though I had just run a marathon.

There was that time my husband hugged me in the kitchen. "Whoa! Why is your heart beating so fast? Is it because you're near me?" Then finally one night after experiencing many rapid heartbeats and a swollen abdomen, I could not sleep at all. I sat on my couch for three hours having difficulty breathing. It was hard just to maneuver myself from one position to the other. Finally, I managed to get myself off the couch and went in to wake my husband. I told him what was happening. He originally wanted to take me to the emergency room right then. I didn't feel it was life-threatening after dealing with this for several weeks already, so we agreed to wait until the morning after the kids left for school to head to the hospital.

The following morning, right after the kids left, we went to a local hospital. I didn't know what was happening and if it was something serious, I would just seek better care at a better hospital. Luckily, only a few people were in the

E.R. at the time, so we briefly sat down and waited before being called in. They put me in a room, took my history, and started an IV so they could administer a diuretic to reduce the amount of fluid in me. I must have had to unhook myself from all the wires attached to me at least five times to go to the bathroom. After several hours, the hospital decided to admit me. They didn't know what was causing my heart rate to be so high so they wanted to run more tests. This time I was given a private room with a bathroom. But take it from me. Something's always gotta give. You can have a great room with great meals and such, but the hospital staff is lacking in their medical expertise. Or you can have top-notch doctors with the best equipment and brains to help you, but the room will suck as well as the food. Cut yourself and need stitches? I'll take option one. Need open heart surgery, please take me to the latter.

The hospitalist there was nice, and she seemed efficient but the cardiologist on staff there, a freaking joke. My cardiologist was not affiliated with this hospital so all he could do was be following this Doofus. Then there was the hospital equipment, the pulse oximeter, in particular. I like to wear dark nail polish. I've had deep red and dark brown nails when I've been at the hospital where I had my surgeries. This time, they were dark as well since Halloween was approaching. I've never encountered a problem. But this time now, over and over, the nurses tried to get an accurate reading of the amount of oxygen in my blood. When they couldn't, they blamed my nail polish color. "We are going to have to remove the color from one finger, just one."

"Nope, not happening. I just had them done and even if you remove just one, do you think that I'd be fine with that? That will look stupid!" I barked back. Their response was even dumber.

"We can try your toe." My toes were the same color as my nails.

"If my finger won't work, what makes you think my toe will?" This went on for two days.

Oh yeah, I was there for a week. There's a medication to regulate your heart rate. The Doofus just couldn't figure out the right dosage. He would order a higher dosage causing the nurses to run into my room and check on me because my heart rate would drop significantly. Then he would order a lower dosage and the palpitations were off the chart.

On the third day, my nurse for the day walked in. I did not care for her. She appeared to be a few years older than my Gianna but was a little bitch. I have much respect for nurses and what they do daily but not this one. She tells me that they must get an accurate reading from the oximeter and my polish must come off. To this day, I think she took pleasure in telling me that because she knew I was against it. Anyway, I like to think that nurses are intelligent individuals. So what she told me baffled me. "I will take it off on your toe. You can wear hospital socks so no one will even know because they won't be able to see your feet. We don't have nail polish remover here so I will use an alcohol prep to remove it." I just looked at her like she had two heads. Was she for real? First, will the sock even fit over the oximeter? Secondly, I'm no nurse, but I'm pretty sure alcohol preps do not take off nail polish! But at this point, I just wanted to leave and wanted to prove this little bitch wrong, so I agreed. As a the result, the color did not come off my toe. All she managed to do was remove the shine off my toe. So now my foot had four shiny toes and one dull one. Asshole!

For the rest of the week, my heart rate went up, and then it went way down while the Doofus played with the dosage. At least the avocado toast was good. I ended up being there for a week. On the final day, the Doofus walks in and I kid you not, throws his hands in the air. "I give up. I don't know what else to do." Never in my whole medical encounters with any medical professional, nurse, general practitioner, or specialist, have I heard those words. I'm not into giving someone a bad reputation so I refrained from mentioning his name, hence Doofus. But, I lost the tiny bit of respect I had for this man at that moment. "What doctor says that?" To this day, when someone asks for a cardiologist's recommendation on social media and someone else recommends him, I cringe. I don't go as far as to comment back but if it is someone I hold dear to me, you best believe they are getting a private message from me! So anyway, I told my family what was happening and the next thing I knew, I was being transferred down to the hospital where I had my surgeries. Here I go in the ambulance again. But at least now I knew I'd be taken care of. I passed that stupid nurse in the hallway. I try to be classy and not trashy, so rather than give her the finger-like I wanted to, I blew her a kiss as they wheeled me by.

I got to the next hospital and met my nurse right away. I would only be with her for a little while as they were changing shifts soon. She was great however and pretty too. She was nice and down to earth. I immediately liked her and hoped that if I stayed here for a day or two she would be my nurse. After I got settled, my parents left, (it had been a long day for them) I kissed my husband and told him to take off too. We still had kids to take care of and they needed at least one parent home. He said goodbye and when he left, I sobbed. I didn't know what was going on with me but I needed this to be over already.

The nurse shift was about to happen, and I got nervous. What I didn't need right now was some nasty-ass nurse. My heart rate was high enough. I didn't need more stress. Soon thereafter, a young nurse walked in. She introduced herself and was sweet. Thank God, I thought as she gently took my vitals. My bed was the first bed when you walked into the room, not the one next to the window.

The view was that of the river and bridge. It was nice to look at. My nurse whispers to me, that my roommate is being discharged tomorrow and that if I am still here, that side will be mine. I smiled and thanked her.

The next day, I had a day nurse who was ok. She wasn't as friendly as the previous nurse but wasn't nasty either. My roommate was discharged that morning. My nurse told me that there is an order in my file to be moved over to the window side. I smiled again. "Thanks, Dinah." Dinah was the nighttime nurse from yesterday. So once the roommate left, that side was cleaned and I was moved. I immediately opened the shade and let the sun in. At least there something should shine from all this.

Although my cardiologist stayed in the office to see patients, he had colleagues that saw the hospital patients and they all worked as a team. My doctor wanted a Congenital Heart Disease doctor to examine me as well. That morning, that doctor along with his partner came to see me. They listened to my heartbeat and took notes. He was an older gentleman but had a pleasant and professional mannerisms about himself. Upon leaving my room, he squeezed my ankle. "Don't worry. We'll figure this out. You won't leave here until we do." I knew then that I was in the right place and felt confident now in the hands of the medical staff overseeing my case.

As I mentioned, Halloween was approaching, and I felt terrible that I wasn't going to be with Mia. Luckily, one of the mothers from my Girl Scout troop offered to take her trick or treating with them. Her daughter was in the same class as my daughter as well and they were friends. That eased my mind somewhat. I needed Mia to be happy in all this. At least my older two could understand and function without me. For Mia, not having her mom around at eight years old was tough. My troop also made cards for me and they were dropped off by my husband. He brought them to the hospital, and I taped them around the window. The troop parents sent me flowers and a teddy bear which I put on the windowsill in the middle. I made my little area a little more cheerful. My husband walked into my room just as I finished decorating. "Looks nice. I guess you're planning on staying a while."

"Let's hope not," I said with a frown. "I just want to look at something cheery from my bed." He looked at me all seriously. "It's Friday Stacy. If they don't make moves today, you are

258

probably here for the weekend no matter what. Nothing is happening on a Sunday or Saturday." Just then, the physician's assistant, Jeff walked in. "Stacy, we'd like to do an MRI of the chest on you. It can give us some more clues and maybe answers to this predicament. I put in an order for you."

"Will this happen today?" I wanted to get out of here no matter how nice my window looked now. "That depends. There are orders for other patients and the department has to be available immediately if they get an emergency. Each test is an hour. They can only do so many in a day." I was hopeful for the test but concerned it would not happen today. "Is the test done over the weekend as well?" "No. You would then have to wait for Monday. I'll try my best to get you in." Jeff walked out. I looked at my husband and did the sign of the cross. He looked at me and said, "Hey, at least we're moving forward with a plan now."

"Yeah, but to be hospitalized for nine days

before performing the test is ridiculous. This couldn't have been done already at the other hospital? Oh wait, a Doofus was running the show." That doctor, not that he is even worthy of that title, really sucked. I feel for anyone having him as a cardiologist.

That evening, my husband left for home when my dinner arrived. It had been a long day and our kids needed him home. He kissed me goodbye. "I love you," I said as I began to eat. Every time someone left, my heart felt a pang of sadness. Not long after I finished the last bite of my meal, Jeff rushed into my room. I looked at him with surprise. "You're still here?" "Stacy, I got you in for the test! But we have to go right now! The technician who does the test is doing me a favor. It's almost the end of his shift but he's willing to do it if we go right now!" "Let's do this!" I shouted. Jeff started unhooking me from all the machines. "There's no time to call a transporter. I'm taking you myself." Once I was free from all the wires, he had me walk to a gurney in the hallway. "Hop on, we're going for a ride!" What I didn't know was that the Radiology department was on the other side of the hospital. I was on that gurney for at least fifteen minutes, whizzing by everyone. I think we came pretty close to knocking some patients over. There is a walkway over a street that connects two buildings. The Radiology department was in the other building. The walkway is made of glass so I could see the traffic below. It must have been some sight to look up from a car and see me being pushed on a gurney as fast as someone running. I didn't know those things could move that fast! I got to the Radiology department finally and Jeff looked like he needed a cardiologist himself! He was panting and full of sweat. "I'm going home now. Good luck Stacy." He left and I was left with two women and a man.

I've had MRIs before but never the chest. This type of MRI sucked compared to the others I've had. For one, it's longer than most. Secondly, you're exposed. I had to remove my gown and be topless. The staff had to put wires on my chest. This involved lifting my breasts and touching them all over. Having females do it is one thing, but with a man doing it as well, I felt very vulnerable. It was humiliating. I just told myself to think of the big picture. This could be the answer to my issue and get me home sooner to my family. Once I was done, I put on a fresh gown and one of the female techs offered to take me back. "You will be here forever if you wait for transport." So, we headed out.

Moments later, the tech gets a call on her phone. "I'm taking the patient back to her room," she says. "Ok, well, I guess he'll find out." She started laughing. I got back to my room and climbed into my bed. Jeff showed up five minutes later, panting and sweating again. "There you are!" I looked at him like he was crazy. "Why are you still here? And did you just work out?" He catches his breath and tells me that he stuck around because he knew that it would take another hour for transport to get me, so he went back for me. Little did he know, I had a ride! Jeff told me the results won't be ready until Monday morning but at least the test was done. It would either confirm what the problem is or rule out certain abnormalities. "Now, I'm going home," he smirked.

So, the weekend went by pretty uneventfully. My family just came to visit. I just ate and watched TV. I occasionally went for short walks around the cardiac wing to get some exercise. What else was there to do? My test results were read first thing on Monday. The doctors came to see me later that morning.

"We believe based on all the findings, that the electrical signals being passed through your heart are being disrupted resulting in arrhythmias or irregular heartbeats. As you are aware, we have been testing different dosage amounts to regulate your heart rhythm. We believe we now have the correct dosage. So now you will go home, take the medicine as prescribed, and follow up with your cardiologist in about two weeks." I didn't know whether to be relieved or disgusted. I was glad they found the issue and had a cure for it, but it took two weeks away from my normal life and disrupted everyone else's around me, to only prescribe a medication? The medication I was already taking, just had to figure out the correct dosage? With that, I was discharged the following day. I took down all of my cards, said goodbye to the staff, and was on my way back to being a wife and mom.

My troop was scheduled for a meeting the following day. My co-leader picked up my daughter. I was staying home so I could rest. No one, not even my daughter knew I was planning on stopping by the meeting, even just for a few minutes because I missed their little faces and to thank them for the joy they brought me in the hospital. Why rest? That was all I did for the past two weeks! I had no restrictions on driving. The only difference now from before being admitted is that now I was on daily medication and needed a pedicure. When I got to the library, the meeting was in full swing. I opened the door and yelled

"Surprise!" My little ladies all smiled, ran up

to me, and hugged me, except for my daughter who looked puzzled. Laughing)

Chapter 14

(2020) "A Whole New World"

Once home, I took my pills on the regular. My stomach was no longer extended but I could still feel my heart race from time to time. I made an appointment to see my cardiologist. Upon examination he referred me to one of his colleagues at work who was not only a cardiologist but specialized in electrophysiology. This doctor sat with me and showed me the interruptions of my heart rhythm on my electrocardiogram report. He discussed a procedure he does as an outpatient called an ablation and that I was a candidate for it. Basically, it's a procedure where a catheter moves up your groin towards your heart to burn the electrical signals that are causing the abnormalities. I was concerned and frightened. "So basically, it's like a catheterization, only longer? "I am awake and can feel some pain? The doctor told me there should be no pain, just a pinch from the local anesthesia. Then I may have some discomfort or soreness following the procedure. His explanation got worse. "There's no guarantee that I will have success in finding the signal. "What do you mean?" I asked. I had a flashback to when they wanted to put that stent in me years ago. That was all for nothing also. "The signals are sporadic, so they are not always in an abnormal way when we're doing the procedure. You don't want me scarring healthy viable ones. It's a chance we take, unfortunately." I wanted to scream but yet what choice did I have?

Besides, with everything else I've been through this is just another battle I'd face. "Let's do it and hope for the best," I replied as once again I made praying hands.

The procedure was not too bad, as promised, I only felt a tiny pinch. In the recovery room, they brought me lunch, I had a television and my husband to chat with. The nurse said I had to walk a bit to loosen up my groin and get the blood flowing. My husband was instructed to walk with me since I still had some leftover anesthesia in me. Upon walking around in recovery, I saw Jeff. "Hey Jeff!" Jeff jumped so high I'd thought he'd pee himself! (laughing) At first, I wasn't sure he recognized me. He looked confused. Plus, he probably encounters so many patients on a daily basis. However, he did recognize me. He spoke after catching his breath from his scare. "Stacy! Good to see you! But why are you back? Oh no! Don't tell me something else happened." I explained why I was there, and he wished me well. His patient was waiting, and my nurse was wondering why it was taking me so long to do a lap around the floor. I got back to my area of the recovery room. The doctor who performed the ablation came to see me. "We were successful Stacy. The electrical signal jumped right out at me. There may be others but this one was definitely contributing to your discomfort. Most of your symptoms should be alleviated after this. If it continues, please come see me. Otherwise, follow up with your doctor. Good luck to you." With that, I said my goodbyes, finished in the recovery room and went home. Luckily, the procedure was in February of 2020 and not after. It would have been extremely difficult to plan for any medical procedures after this and who knew the entire world was about to shut down.

The Coronavirus or more currently known as Covid-19, shut everyone down. For the first time, I witnessed doors to stores, restaurants and more being closed. My kids could not attend school and even my oldest daughter who was seven hours away had to return home. While everyone was taking extreme precautions, I had to take it even further. I had an underlying condition that absolutely could not come in contact with the virus. What made matters worse, is that I needed a follow up with the cardiologist after the ablation, a few weeks later. I mentioned I had it done in February. Pretty much everything shut down the week of March 16, 2020, right when I was due to go back. I was petrified to walk out of my house, let alone go to the doctor's office. A telehealth visit was mentioned at some point. What the hell was the doctor staring at me through a computer screen going to do for me. "Here, Stacy, lean your chest toward the screen so I can take a listen?" C'mon! I'm all for new technology and appreciate how advanced medicine has come but some things must remain exactly how they are. I decided it was better to take my chances and assume my heart is functioning well rather than risk going for a visit and contracting Covid. Besides, my 2020 curse already had happened. I needed an ablation. So I continued on as normal, staying in my home and just going in the backyard if I needed some outside air. I was always busy anyhow.

Because we were always home now, the house constantly got messy and needed to be cleaned. My kids were forced to have school virtually, so I had to help them with their lessons. The girl scout meetings were put on a hold for a bit, however. Parents, myself included, had it hard enough already, to get their kids to log on to a Google Meet or a Zoom meeting. My heart condition put me at such a risk that my daughter and son had to do the food shopping for us. They had to wear masks and gloves. My daughter often complained about getting "chewed "out by a stranger in the supermarket for not walking in the correct direction of the arrows. There was a shortage of hand sanitizer, Lysol and toilet paper. The first two I could see. Ya gotta get rid of those germs. But toilet paper? (laughing) It definitely was a rough time.

Every day and all day, whether it was on social media, tv or the radio, someone was talking about the virus. The death toll was definitely a downer. I eventually stopped listening to the radio and watching the news. When ordering new clothing, I would order a new mask too like I was ordering matching socks. It was sort of fun in a weird way. We needed different size masks too. Mia needed a kid size while the rest of us needed adults. My husband still had to go to work every day. I was so afraid to be near him because of his whereabouts during the day. He was careful as much as he could be but you never knew. My parents couldn't visit and that was terrible too since I was used to seeing them often. The kids missed them and vice versa.

When the vaccine came out, it was hard to find an appointment even though I was eligible since I was compromised. One of my girl scout moms and a dear friend, pulled some strings and got me in. I had my vaccine which eased my mind a little. Once we all became used to a daily routine of having many things virtually, I began to hold virtual meetings for the troop. Of course, the girls preferred having meetings in person, but it just wasn't possible. I was afraid I would lose some of them over this.

Eventually, situations improved. The death toll and hospital admissions started to decline. Businesses started re-opening. The kids were going to be back in school that fall. We planned a vacation for that summer to take the kids away.

All we had to do was wear a mask in the plane and inside the hotel. The vacation went well. It was desperately needed after being cooped up for so long. But Covid did have its strong points.

We grew as a family from it. We spent quality time with one another that we probably would not have if we didn't have to stay home Especially with my eldest. Her college switched to remote learning so she could continue her education from home and not return to campus. It was nice having her home after her not being around for the past year. But, her graduation from college was virtual so that sucked. Prior to Covid, I was looking forward to the day I'd see her walk across the stage and get her college degree. Now she is in grad school and her college is twenty minutes away!

As I write this, it is now 2022. My fingers are crossed. Every now and then I feel a pain in my heart. Does the two-year curse live on or is it simply my mind playing tricks on me? I saw the cardiologist a few weeks ago followed by an echo. It took a few days for the results to come in. I had a follow-up appointment to discuss the findings. There were none. Nothing had changed since my last test. "But what am I feeling?" I had asked the doctor. He looked up from his computer. "I am not sure what you are feeling. The echo came out fine which is a good thing. However, I do want to address the symptoms you are experiencing. I'd like you to follow up with the congenital heart disease doctor for further evaluation." So, I did just that. This doctor was the one that squeezed my ankle in the hospital and helped solve that issue. He performed his own echo to look at additional images. He also didn't find anything. He ordered a heart monitor for me to wear for three weeks. "Three weeks! It's July, can't this wait? What if I want to go to the beach? Again, you're probably wondering where my priorities are. But I am just tired of always being held back for my heart. "Wear it and when you want to go swimming, you can take it off for a few hours." I am wearing the heart monitor now as I type this. What will the results be? Will there be more to this story? For my sake, I hope my story continues on in life but not where there's anything to say related to health. I have finally decided to let it all go, hence writing this book. If you remember anything from reading it, remember this. Laughter is key. Without it, life is simply boring. Laughter can uplift someone's spirits in the darkest moments. Even in the worst of moments, try to find it. Don't take life so seriously. No one gets out alive anyway. This is my story.